ACUPUNCTURE: CURE OF MANY DISEASES

Second Edition

BY

FELIX MANN

MB, BChir (Cambridge)
LMCC
Founder and President (1959–1980) of The Medical Acupuncture Society
First President of The British Medical Acupuncture Society (1980)
Co-ordinator of The Acupuncture, Scientific and Clinical Advisory Group

FOREWORD BY
ALDOUS HUXLEY

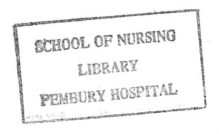
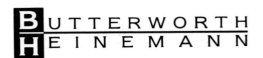
BUTTERWORTH
HEINEMANN

Butterworth-Heinemann Ltd
Linacre House, Jordan Hill, Oxford OX2 8DP

 PART OF REED INTERNATIONAL BOOKS

OXFORD LONDON BOSTON
MUNICH NEW DELHI SINGAPORE SYDNEY
TOKYO TORONTO WELLINGTON

First Published 1971
Revised Reprint 1972
Reprinted 1973
Reprinted 1975
Reprinted 1980
Second Edition 1992

Spanish edition published by Editorial Pomaire S.A. 1972
Dutch edition published by Driehoek 1973
Finnish edition published by Tammi 1974
German edition published by Karl F. Haug 1976
Italian edition published by Mondazzi 1980
Swedish edition published by A.B. Arcanum 1984

© Felix Mann 1971, 1992

British Library Cataloguing in Publication Data
Mann, Felix
  Acupuncture: Cure of Many Diseases. –
  2Rev.ed
  I. Title
  615.8

ISBN 0 7506 0700 9

Library of Congress Cataloguing in Publication Data
Mann, Felix.
  Acupuncture: cure of many diseases/by Felix Mann; Foreword by
  Aldous Huxley. – 2nd ed.
  p. cm.
  ISBN 0 7506 0700 9
  1. Acupuncture.   I. Title.
  [DNLM: 1. Acupuncture – popular works. WB 369 M281ab]
  RM184.M338 1992
  615.8′92–dc20   92–20085
                                                             CIP

Printed and bound in Great Britain by
Biddles Ltd, Guildford and King's Lynn

FOREWORD
by Aldous Huxley

That a needle stuck into one's foot should improve the functioning of one's liver is obviously incredible. It can't be believed because, in terms of currently accepted physiological theory 'it makes no sense'. Within our system of explanation there is no reason why the needle-prick should be followed by an improvement of liver function. Therefore, we say, it can't happen.

The only trouble with this argument is that, as a matter of empirical fact, it does happen. Inserted at precisely the right point, the needle in the foot regularly affects the function of the liver.

What should we do about events which, by all the rules, ought not to occur, but which nevertheless occur?

Two courses are open to us. We can either shut our eyes to the queer embarrassing data in the hope that, if we don't look at them, they will go away and leave us in peace. Or alternatively we can accept them—accept them for the time being as inexplicable anomalies, while doing our best to modify current theory in such a way that it will 'save the appearances'—*all* the appearances including those queer events that now seem to be outside the pale of explicability.

Herbert Spencer's idea of tragedy (in T. H. Huxley's words) was 'a beautiful Generalisation murdered by an ugly Fact'. The author of the Synthetic Philosophy died many years ago; but his scholastic soul goes marching along, and the tendency to prefer the high hallowed generalisation to the low, odd, presumptuous datum is still to be met with even in the most respectable scientific circles. From telepathy to acupuncture, queer facts get ignored by the very people whose business it is to investigate them—get ignored because they fail to fit into any of the academic pigeonholes and do not suffer themselves to be explained in terms of accredited theories.

It was through the Jesuit missionaries that the first accounts of acupuncture reached the West. These early reports were glowing but vague, and it was not until 1928 that a full and accurate account of this curious branch of Chinese medicine became available to European readers. In that year Soulié de Morant returned from China and published his first treatise on the subject. Today several hundreds of European doctors practise the ancient science and art of acupuncture in conjunction with the science and art of Western medicine. International Congresses of Acupuncture are periodically convened (the most recent of them was held at the University of Clermont-Ferrand), and it is reported that Soviet physicians have begun to take a lively interest in the subject. In England, I am happy to say, we have the author of this volume; though recently a few more have taken it up, or have used it as an adjunct to ordinary medicine. Let us hope that he will succeed in persuading his colleagues and the public that the method produces good results, even though it may not, for the moment, and in terms of Western science (1961), make sense.

To the Chinese, of course, it made perfectly good sense. In the normally healthy organism, they maintained, there is a continuous circulation of energy. Illness is at once the result and the cause of a derangement of this circulation. Where energy fails to circulate as it should, vital organs may suffer from a deficiency, or a disturbing excess of the life-force. Acupuncture is effective because it re-directs and normalises the flow of energy. This is possible because (as a matter of empirical fact) the limbs, trunk and head are lined with invisible 'meridians', related in some way to the various organs of the body. On these meridians are located certain peculiarly sensitive points. A needle inserted at one of these points will exert an influence on the organ related to the meridian on which the point lies. By pricking at a number of carefully selected points, the skilled acupuncturist reestablishes the normal circulation of energy and brings his patient back to health.

'All very fine,' we are tempted to say. 'But it still makes no sense.' After reading the proceedings of the most recent Congress of Acupuncture, I suspect that, after all, it may make a little sense. Experimenters report that they have succeeded, by means of delicate electrical measuring instruments, in tracing the course of the Chinese 'meridians', and that relatively large changes of electrical state are recorded when strategic points are pricked with a needle. So perhaps, in the end, the anomalous appearances of acupuncture can be saved even by *our* theories. Meanwhile, the fact remains that there are many pathological symptoms, on which the old Chinese methods work very well. For the patient whose only wish is to get well as quickly as possible, this is all that matters.

This foreword was originally written by Aldous Huxley for my first book, *Acupuncture: The Ancient Chinese Art of Healing*, which is a semi-technical book. I have now transferred his foreword to this book, which is written for the layman. This is commensurate with Aldous Huxley's own writings, which though dealing with difficult subjects were written in a style readable by all.

PREFACE

Acupuncture is a system of medicine whereby some diseases intractable to orthodox treatment may be cured or alleviated. Anyone who reads the long list of diseases that may be helped by acupuncture (in Chapter X or the statistics at the end of the book) may think the list rather presumptuous, as if acupuncture were to be regarded as a general panacea. It should be realised, however, that acupuncture is not a single drug, such as penicillin, which is therapeutically applicable to only a limited variety of infections. Acupuncture is, on the contrary, a whole system of medicine which encompasses many dysfunctions of the body – hence the title of this book.

Parts of this book were written some thirty years ago, soon after I had started practising acupuncture. Some parts were written a few years later. In those days, as far as I know, I was the first and the only doctor to practise solely acupuncture in this country.

Naturally there was opposition, of a polite variety, from the medical establishment: 'My grandmother sat on a drawing pin and was cured of her imaginary illness'. Luckily I had the enthusiasm of youth to overcome this; the evangelical zeal that a new method of medicine can arouse; the wish to do something that did not only regard a human being as something material; the constant support of my mother and that of my patients who were open-minded enough to judge by results.

This enthusiasm, without which it would have been impossible to survive in the early days, had its drawbacks. There was the tendency to think that the achievements of acupuncture were greater than they really were and that acupuncture was more universally applicable than it really is. In those days, as will be apparent to the reader, I actually enthusiastically believed in the traditional Chinese concepts and theories of medicine. Today, as the reader of the scientific section of my

Textbook of Acupuncture might notice, my ideas are largely. different.

When reading through this, the Second Edition, I realised how great this change had been. Some of the things I read made me alternately blush, squirm in my seat or made my hair stand on end. In a few sections, however, I think I was cleverer then than now.

Nevertheless I have left the book essentially as it is for it describes traditional Chinese acupuncture as seen through the eyes of a Western believer. Now, after practising solely acupuncture for over thirty years, my results are better than in the early days, but as I am no longer an evangelist I am less starry-eyed about the statistics.

Although this book highlights the virtues of acupuncture and mentions some of the failures of orthodox Western medicine, let no-one imagine that I under-rate ordinary medicine. Indeed, if my practice were in the country I would combine both schools, using whichever method was better in a particular patient or disease. However, since I am in central London, I tend to specialise in those diseases where acupuncture is the better method of treatment combining (which will not be apparent from this book) the acupuncture with Western physiology, pathology, diagnostic methods and, if appropriate, ordinary drugs.

I would like to thank Ronald Fuller who took on the none too easy task of correcting the text of my original manuscript. I was lucky to find the medical artist Sylvia Treadgold, who has the gift not only of drawing good anatomical and technical illustrations but has also created the cartoons to enliven and highlight the difficult parts of the text.

A full bibliography and acknowledgements are in my more comprehensive book, Textbook of Acupuncture.

The Second Edition contains two new chapters. One on Strong Reactors, as the correct dosage of treatment is the secret of success. The other on the 'liver' which is the point of departure for the treatment of many diverse conditions ranging from migraine to dysmenorrhoea.

LONDON, W.1.   FELIX MANN
1992

CONTENTS

Doctors who wish to study acupuncture are welcome to write to me. Several times a year I hold practical courses which are similar to teaching ward rounds at medical school. These courses were started in 1962 and have been attended by a thousand doctors in forty countries. Since 1963 I have also organised an annual acupuncture symposium for these doctors.

GENERAL THEORY

After qualifying as a doctor at Cambridge University and Westminster Hospital, I decided to go abroad. I had gained a knowledge of orthodox medicine in England but I wanted to explore further, to see how much the practice in other countries might contribute to that knowledge. Among the places I visited was Strasbourg, and it was here that I happened on a method of healing almost unknown at that time in England.

A friend of mine in Strasbourg developed acute appendicitis, for which of course the orthodox treatment would have been an immediate operation. This she refused to consider. Instead, she asked for her own special doctor, who cured her by the simple but surprising method of sticking a needle into the skin below her knee. Within fifteen minutes the nausea, the pain and muscular rigidity of the abdomen completely disappeared nor was there any recurrence of these symptoms. She retains her appendix to this day.

Such was my first introduction to Acupuncture, an ancient Chinese system of medicine in which needles are used for the cure of disease.

The prick of the needle at certain precisely defined points on the skin stimulates specific nerves, which transmit electrical impulses to the spinal cord and lower centres of the brain and thence to the diseased area (Fig. 1). Nerves are supplied to every part of the body, no matter how small, and every inch of it is under the direct or indirect control of one or a group of nerves. They control nearly all processes going on in the body. When stimulated, some nerves will increase the movement of the intestines, others retard it; some will increase, others decrease, the flow of the digestive juices; and the same is true of the increase or decrease in the rate of the heart, the expansion or contraction of blood-vessels, the flow of tears, the tone of the muscles, the secretion of hormones, the rate of growth and so on. The nervous system can be

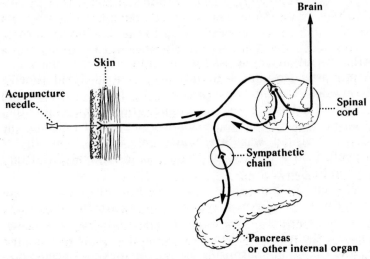

Fig. 1. The nerves along which an impulse travels, from the needle to the diseased organ or part of the body—simplified.

compared to the electronic control apparatus of some complex machine, like a telephone exchange or an automatic pilot. The art of acupuncture depends on knowing precisely which nerve to stimulate in a given disease. It sounds as simple as knowing which keys to press on a typewriter in order to spell your own name. In fact, however, a considerable amount of knowledge is needed before acupuncture can be practised satisfactorily.

You might call it a 'self-regulating' system of medicine, for the nerve-passages stimulated by the needle are the very ones the body itself uses to regulate its several physiological processes. If, for example, there were not some increase in the movement of the stomach and intestines and the secretion of digestive juices at the same time as one has a meal, everything one ate would remain in the stomach undigested. This increased activity of stomach, intestines and digestive juices happens chiefly because the nerves supplying these organs are stimulated, first by the sight of food and then by its taste and presence within the body. In acupuncture these same nerves can be directly stimulated by way of a branch of the nerve network going to the skin. Some of these nerves go to the skin near the digestive organs, others run a more distant course to the various limbs.

But it is unusual for the stomach to increase the flow of the digestive juices unless there is work for them to do; and in the same way, it is unusual for the stimulation of a stomach acupuncture point to produce them if they are not needed. This is how acupuncture is self-regulating and why, if it is backed by a thorough medical knowledge, it is probably the safest system of medicine in existence.

The ancient Chinese described the flow of nervous energy in the body as 'Qi'*—the energy of life: what we would call a wave of electrical depolarisation spreading along the nerve. They called the principal nerve endings 'acupuncture points' and the main course of a similar group of nerve endings (possibly related to dermatomes) 'meridians'.

To the Chinese a human being was a living unity, a field for the action and interaction of the invisible forces of life. The harmony of these vital powers within him was revealed by the health of the whole body, their disharmony by its disease, their disappearance by its death. So the aim of the Chinese doctor was to correct the imbalance of the vital forces in the body. Once the harmonious interplay of these forces had been restored, the patient himself was able to overcome his weakness.

In the Western world today we all too often tend to picture man as a kind of chemical factory or as a none too reliable machine constantly in need of repair. The invisible and imponderable powers within him, 'spirit', 'life forces', 'soul', we separate from the physical machine. If they are not

* Pronounced chee as in cheese.

mere creatures of our own fantasy, they belong to the mysterious and ill-defined provinces of the theologian or psychiatrist. So when something goes wrong with any part of the machine, the doctor investigates it rather as a garage technician investigates a badly functioning car. When the fault is found, spare parts are supplied. So, if the patient is diabetic, the missing insulin is replaced; if he is anaemic, he needs more iron; if he suffers from some infection the bacteria which cause it are killed off, or he may be immunised against certain infections. The patient is 'well' again—until another nut or bolt in the machine needs renewing.

Modern medical researchers use all the resources of science in their efforts to discover the biochemical processes going on

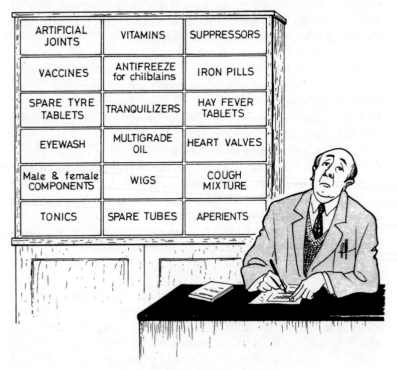

ARTIFICIAL JOINTS	VITAMINS	SUPPRESSORS
VACCINES	ANTIFREEZE for chilblains	IRON PILLS
SPARE TYRE TABLETS	TRANQUILIZERS	HAY FEVER TABLETS
EYEWASH	MULTIGRADE OIL	HEART VALVES
Male & female COMPONENTS	WIGS	COUGH MIXTURE
TONICS	SPARE TUBES	APERIENTS

Fig. 2. The mechanistic doctor.

in the human body—as intricate and laborious a task as trying to find an unknown quantity of needles in innumerable haystacks. As soon as he discovers a broken link in the chain of chemical processes, the doctor replaces it with some synthetic drug, which his patient may well have to go on taking throughout his entire span of life. The drug is usually a temporary replacement. It is not a cure.

If a doctor thinks in this mechanistic way, he will see a patient as needing the equivalents of fuel, spare parts, lubricants or emulsifying agents (Fig. 2). But in the East the doctor tends to think of his patient as an organic being with the powers of life within him, who can become a harmonious whole in health and vitality without needing constant replacements for his body. Mind and body form a living unity and cannot be treated as if they were separate. A human being is more than an aggregate of physical substances and chemical processes. Life is something that exists in its own right.

Both the Eastern and Western approaches have their value for the sick patient. One day, I hope, they can be combined and doctors will be able to think both mechanistically and in terms of the life forces. We in the West have long taken it for granted that our methods are the best; but the ancient wisdom of the East can make a no less important contribution to medicine.

'The root of acupuncture is in the spirit. . .'
'The human spirit is endowed from heaven. The physical energy is endowed from the earth.'

(Jia Yi Jing, Vol. I, Ch. 1)

II

THE ACUPUNCTURE POINTS

In all diseases, whether physical or mental, there are tender areas at certain points on the surface of the body, which disappear when the illness is cured.

These are so-called acupuncture* points.

In some cases they will be spontaneously painful. When, for example, a patient suffers from a frontal headache, he will feel pain in the area where the skull joins with the back of the neck, a point known as gall bladder 20 (Fig. 3). In

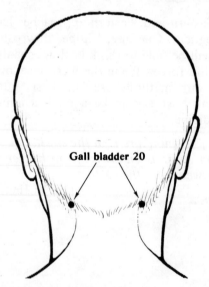

Fig. 3. The area near gall bladder 20 is often tender in frontal headaches.

* Acus is the Latin for a needle.

other cases, however, these points are only tender under pressure, so that there would be no pain at all at, say, gall bladder 20 until pressure was applied. To this category belong the many points just above the ankle. Women in particular are unaware how tender this area is unless it is pressed. Thirdly there is the type of acupuncture point where there is no tenderness at all, even under pressure, so that they can only be found by the hand of the experienced physician.

The doctor looking for an acupuncture point will, in the simplest of instances, discover a little nodule, like the fibrositic rheumatic nodules often present at the back of the neck, in the shoulders or in the lumbar area (Fig. 4 upper).

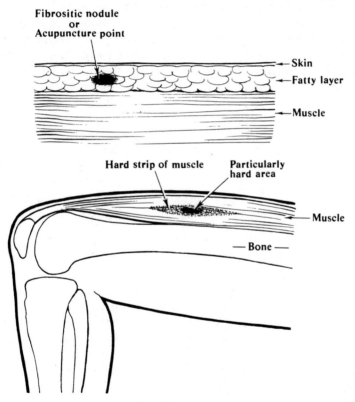

Fig. 4. Two varieties of acupuncture points.

But in many cases instead of the nodule the examining finger may find a strip of tense muscle within a group of muscles with a particularly hard and indurated area (Fig. 4 lower). Sometimes there is an area which is slightly swollen or discoloured. In the most difficult cases the point cannot be found without a knowledge of its exact anatomical position.

Some people use an electrical instrument to measure the electrical skin resistance or impedance. The theory is that, since the impedance is reduced at the acupuncture points, they can in this way be easily and accurately discovered. I have myself tried three of these and one experimental apparatus, but have found that the electrical resistance both in living bodies and cadavers varies in so many places, not only at the acupuncture points but at thousands of others, that to me such apparatus is of little use. Formerly a number of doctors, including myself, hoped it might be possible to locate the acupuncture points electrically (Fig. 5). If, though, acupuncture works via the nervous system, the construction of the apparatus would have to take its special electrical properties into account.

As mentioned above, the pain at those acupuncture points which are either spontaneously tender or tender under pressure vanishes with the cure of the disease. It makes no difference how the cure has been achieved, whether by acupuncture, ordinary drugs, osteopathic manipulation, homeopathy, hypnosis or the mere passage of time: when the illness ends, so also does the pain.

This at once establishes a causal relationship between disease, physical as well as mental, and the tender variety of acupuncture point.

In one very simple form of acupuncture diagnosis, the patient is examined from head to toes in order to find all the tender points, and hence to deduce the internal disease corresponding to them. Some of these points are known and used for diagnosis in orthodox medicine, though of course the average doctor is unaware that these are acupuncture points. Thus the right shoulder, particularly at point gall bladder 21, may be spontaneously tender in gall bladder disease, bladder 23 in kidney disease and the appendix area near point stomach 26 in appendicitis (Fig. 6).*

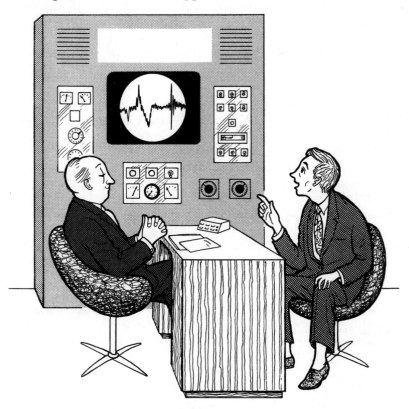

Fig. 5.

The acupuncture points can serve a dual purpose, for not only do they help in the diagnosis of disease but may also conversely be used for its treatment. In this the skin is pierced at the acupuncture point by a fine needle, which is withdrawn usually after the lapse of a few minutes.

* For positions of acupuncture points see: Atlas of Acupuncture.

'When the vision is blurred and the eye does not see, the side of the head is painful, likewise the outer corner of the eye. This is cured by needling the point "Jaw Detested",' (*gall bladder 4*).

(Jia Yi Jing, Vol. XII, Ch. 4)

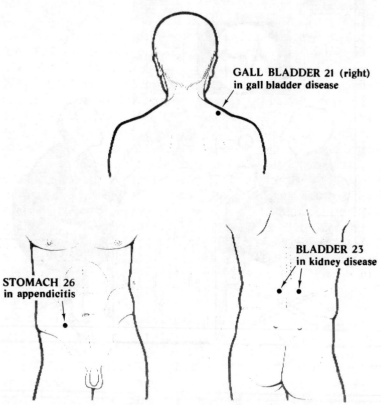

GALL BLADDER 21 (right)
in gall bladder disease

BLADDER 23
in kidney disease

STOMACH 26
in appendicitis

Fig. 6. Some similarities between orthodox medicine and acupuncture.

In one form of acupuncture the points spontaneously tender or those tender under pressure are needled. In other more refined forms, the acupuncturist needles those points where no pain is felt at all, points which are often remote from the seat of the disease and sometimes even on the opposite side of the body.

Occasionally some wholly accidental stimulus to an acupuncture point may cure a disease. I remember when I was at school seeing a couple of boys fighting together on top of a bed. One of them fell down, hitting his forehead at the root of the nose on the iron bedstead, and was immediately cured of the sinus trouble he had suffered from for two or three years. A parallel case is that of a woman with a dull, though mild, headache accompanied by general malaise, which persisted day after day almost unrelieved for some ten years. During these years she had had several blood tests, which involved pricking the skin to reach a vein at the elbow. She soon noticed that, every time her skin was pricked at this point, the headache and malaise instantly disappeared and for a couple of hours she was free of pain. This happened so regularly that she actually began to look forward to her blood tests; but, when she mentioned this to her doctor, tentatively suggesting a connection between the tests and the relief of the headache, he dismissed the idea as nonsensical. When she came to me, I inserted an acupuncture needle into the same place at the elbow. I neither pierced the vein nor drew off any blood; yet the headache at once disappeared, a proof that the cause and effect she had noticed had nothing to do with the loss of blood. She was in time completely cured of her trouble by the additional needling of several other acupuncture points, effective in her particular type of headache.

There are many such apparently accidental correspondences, some of them not generally known. The knock-out points of Judo, for example, are also acupuncture points, which if too strongly stimulated, will cause the subject to collapse in a faint. The Indian points of the Chakras and Nadir similarly correspond to acupuncture points. Deraniyagala, director of the national museums of Ceylon, lists the places which the *mahout*, or Indian elephant boy, prods with a sharp stick to elicit various responses from his elephant* (Fig.7a). Having no personal experience here, I do

* *Some Extinct Elephants, Their Relatives and Two Living Species* (Ceylon National Museum Publication).

not know if these 'Nila' are really acupuncture points, but at least it seems feasible; and perhaps the reason why the African, unlike the Indian, elephant cannot be adequately trained is because the Nila of the African elephant are unknown.

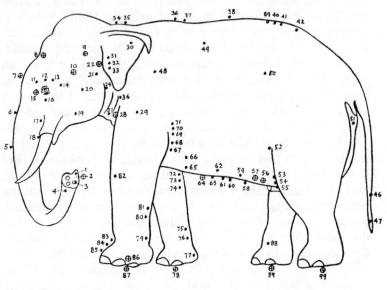

● Nila (nerve centres)

Fig. 7a. Even elephants have acupuncture points.

Some functions of the Nila are as follows:

1. Twists trunk
2. Straightens trunk
3. Frightens
4. Frightens and makes trumpet
5. Frightens, makes trumpet and stops animal
6. Brings under control
23. Bends head
24. Stops animal
25. Rouses, infuriates
35. Benumbs
52. Gets up and runs
55. Turns round
71. Kneels

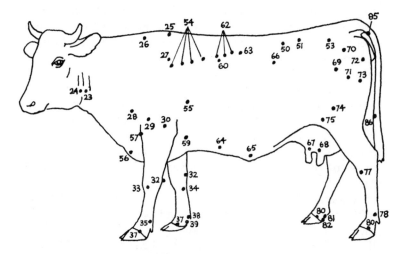

Fig. 7b. Veterinary acupuncture.

Some acupuncture points on the cow are as follows:

23. 'Hot' disease (Hot, cold, wind, damp are traditional Chinese conceptions)
24. Throat swollen, 'wind' disease of throat
26–29. Disease of front legs due to 'wind' and 'damp'
30. Elbow swollen
32. Front of elbow swollen and painful
33, 34. Knee swollen
38. Heel swollen due to 'wind' and 'damp'
50. Loin swollen

51. Kidney 'cold', disease of lumbar area and back legs
55. Liver and gall bladder disease, spleen swollen
57. Heart and lung disease
59. Pain and discomfort in stomach and abdomen
60. Spleen swollen, lack of appetite
62. Spleen and stomach pain
68. Udder swollen, cannot be milked
70–73. Back leg has disease due to 'wind' and 'damp'

The above drawing of a cow shows some of the acupuncture points used by Chinese vets in treating animals–cows, horses, pigs and chickens. It will be noted that the points referred to in the cow, as in man, mention diseases, while those on the elephant deal with movements. Possibly the prodding of a sharp stick at the Nila is only a method of training the elephant.

Several indigenous medical systems in different parts of the world probably correspond to a simple form of acupuncture. Thus some Arabs will cauterise part of the ear with a red-hot poker in treating sciatica, while among the Bantus of South Africa certain healers will scratch small circumscribed areas of the skin and then rub various herbs into them (Fig. 8).

A doctor often has to diagnose mysterious abdominal pains or other symptoms, for which he can find no definite cause. He may therefore suggest to his patient an exploratory operation, in case there is any serious disease present. The surgeon will probably find a spastic colon or mild inflammation of the abdominal lymph nodes or some other not irreversible condition. So he does nothing beyond sewing up the patient and sending him home after a week in hospital. At the follow up a month later, often the patient will tell his doctor that he has been completely cured of his illness, and thank the surgeon for his skilled and timely operation. As for the surgeon, he will probably think in some bewilderment that he must have cured his patient by hypnosis.

One surgeon, who taught me a as medical student, believed that a little air let into the abdomen cured all manner of ills. But is it not possible that the patient was cured because the surgeon's knife stimulated acupuncture points? If so, would it not be much simpler to try acupuncture in such cases and leave to the surgeon only those where surgery is really necessary?

Case History. A patient limped into my consulting room with severe pain in the lower back and leg due to a slipped disc. Physiotherapy, a corset and traction had been tried to no avail. The next attempt on the agenda was a major operation to fuse several vertebrae together with a piece of bone cut from the hip.

I tried acupuncture and the patient was soon cured, but he still has to be careful lifting heavy weights. In some cases where the disc is

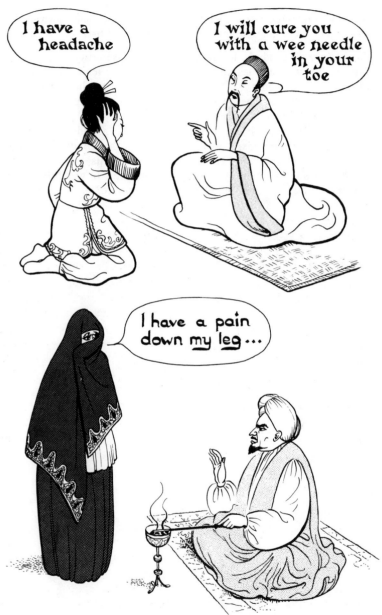

Fig. 8. Not only the Chinese know of acupuncture.

severely prolapsed, an operation may be the only answer, but everything, including acupuncture, should be tried first.

Case History. A lady in her late thirties had severe flooding (called in Chinese 'bursting and leaking disease'). She was anaemic, weak and had often to stay at home. No treatment had helped and her gynaecologist suggested removing her womb at operation. Acupuncture cured her—and she still has her womb today.

If the excessively heavy periods (or having periods non-stop) are caused by large fibroids, a growth or certain other conditions, surgery or radiation is often the best treatment. In the majority of instances flooding is due to a mild dysfunction of the womb or glandular system, which can often be cured or helped by acupuncture.

III

THE MERIDIANS

'The means whereby man is created, the means whereby disease occurs, the means whereby man is cured, the means whereby disease arises: the twelve meridians are the basis of all theory and treatment'.

(Ling Shu, jingbie pian)

In Chinese literature there are descriptions of about a thousand acupuncture points, though there may well be even more than this. Books on the subject are full of accounts of illnesses which can be cured or alleviated by stimulating with a needle one or other of these points. The point called bladder 7 (Fig. 9) for instance, near the top of the head with

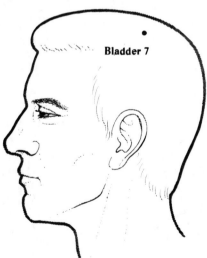

Fig. 9. Acupuncture point bladder 7 may be used in headache. . . .

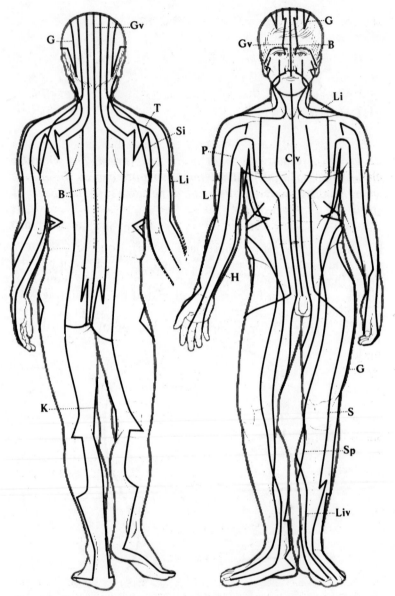

Fig. 10. The 14 important meridians: 12 main meridians, conception vessel (Cv) and governing vessel (Gv).

the picturesque Chinese name of Penetrating Heaven, has an effect on:

'Headache, heaviness of head, glands swollen in the neck, nose blocked, nose bleed, running nose, loss of smell due to catarrh, swelling of the face, neuralgia of the face, breathlessness, chronic bronchitis, dry mouth, thirstiness, epileptic-like convulsions, lack of balance, weak eyesight.'*

Since it is obviously difficult to remember the properties of so large a number of acupuncture points, the Chinese classified them into twelve main groups and a few subsidiary ones. All the acupuncture points belonging to any one of these groups are joined by a line, the Chinese word for which (Jing) means a passage, or nowadays forms part of the word for a nerve. In the West it is called a meridian. The meridians on one side of the body are duplicated by those on the other, just as we have a left as well as a right thumb; but there are two extra meridians, which, since they run up the middle of the body, cannot of course be thus paired.

The twelve main meridians are those of the (Fig. 10):

Full name	Abbreviation	Full name	Abbreviation
lung	L	bladder	B
large intestine	Li	kidney	K
stomach	S	pericardium	P
spleen	Sp	triple warmer	T
heart	H	gall bladder	G
small intestine	Si	liver	Liv

The number of acupuncture points along each of these meridians varies, the heart meridian, for example, having nine

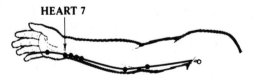

HEART 7

Fig. 11. Heart meridian on right showing its acupuncture points. Heart 1 (under armpit) along arm to heart 9 (at end of little finger).

*Taken from: Textbook of Acupuncture.

points on each side (Fig. 11), while the bladder meridian has sixty-seven. All the acupuncture points on a meridian affect the organ after which they are named.

Case History. One patient of mine suffered from recurrent palpitations and a feeling of pressure across the chest, sometimes during periods of slight mental or physical stress, sometimes for no apparent reason. She easily became breathless walking upstairs, had less than her normal energy and was therefore compelled to rest during the daytime, which meant that she found it harder to get through the day's work.

These symptoms were clearly due to a heart condition; so a needle was inserted at the acupuncture point heart 7 (Fig. 11), called by the Chinese the 'gateway of the spirit', since the spirit was thought to live in the heart. Within a few minutes the symptoms were alleviated and, after half a dozen repetitions of the treatment at fortnightly intervals, the patient was cured.

Clearly this system of classifying a thousand acupuncture points into twelve main (and two extra) meridians is in practice very useful, for if, as in the above instance, a patient has a disease of the heart, one immediately knows which group (meridian) of acupuncture points to use. In this case acupuncture point 7 was used, though any of the other eight points on the heart meridian would have helped, but to a lesser extent. The acupuncture point which has the greatest curative effect in a particular disease or on a particular patient is discussed later in the course of this book.

'The kidney meridian starts at the sole of the foot. . . When it is diseased, the face turns black as charcoal, there is loss of appetite, coughing of blood, harsh panting, a wish to get up when sitting down, the eye cannot see clearly, the heart feels as if suspended.'

(Jia Yi Jing, Vol. II, Ch. 1a)

IV

THE TWELVE SPHERES OF INFLUENCE
IN THE BODY

*'The Thunder God said, "I would like to know about the
course and diseases of meridians, and how through them one
may cure by acupuncture."*
*The Yellow Emperor answered, "The meridian is that
which decides over life and death. Through it the hundred
diseases may be treated".'*

(Jia Yi Jing, Vol. II, Ch. 1a)

The twelve organs and their associated twelve meridians
encompass all parts of the body, with the exceptions of the
head and sense organs, the endocrine glands, the sexual
system, and others. Nevertheless, these can all be successfully
treated, for (though not directly counted among them) they
all belong to one or more than one of the twelve main
meridian groups.

The Main Meridian*

Anything that happens along or near the course of a main
meridian will influence that meridian and the organ which
bears its name.

Case History. A patient who had been troubled with palpitations and
breathlessness for two months, came to consult me, thinking she had a
disease of the heart. In the course of our conversation, she mentioned
that two days before the onset of the symptoms she had sprained her
wrist, and I found that the place where the tenderness was most acute
crossed the heart meridian at acupuncture point 7 (Fig. 11). The
constant irritation at this point over several days had in turn affected
the heart. In this instance the patient was cured of her heart symptoms

*For greater detail see: Textbook of Acupuncture.

by treating the sprained wrist rather than by a direct treatment of the heart. The similarity between this case history and that at the end of chapter III, which was concerned with a genuine disease of the heart, should be noted.

Embryological Relationships

When acupuncture points on the kidney meridian are stimulated, they affect not only the kidney but also embryologically related organs, such as the ovary, testicle, uterus, fallopian tube and, to some extent, the adrenal. This is because all these organs, while the human embryo is in the womb of the mother, are formed from more or less the same tissue, and in the same region, as the kidney. This intimate relationship in the embryo is maintained in the adult, at least in so far as kidney acupuncture points are concerned (Fig. 12).

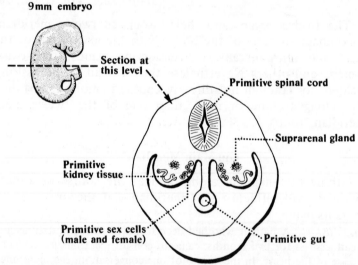

Fig. 12. The kidney, the suprarenal gland, the ovary or testicle originate as neighbours in the embryo.

This, only one among hundreds of embryological relationships, is an example of how the interdependence of different parts of the body can be utilised in acupuncture.

Anatomical and Functional Relationships

In the adult the nose and throat are part of the respiratory system; in the embryo, however, the throat is part of the alimentary tract, from which the nose is split off. As far as acupuncture is concerned, diseases of the nose and throat can usually be treated through lung acupuncture points, the lung being the main respiratory organ. Hence, in this instance, the adult function predominates rather than the embryological relationship described in the previous section. Nasal catarrh, or hay fever, for example, may be treated in this way by using acupuncture point lung 7 (Fig. 13), though as a rule a few accessory points are also needed.

LUNG 7

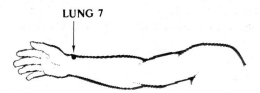

Fig. 13. Nasal catarrh or hay fever may be treated by stimulating acupuncture point lung 7.

Physiological Relationships

The stimulation of one of the fourteen paired acupuncture points on the liver meridian will improve on obvious liver disease, like jaundice; but several other ailments less evidently from this source can also be cured or alleviated, such as:

Migraine, a condition which makes the patient feel nauseated and bilious—and indeed was once known as 'the megrims' or bouts of billiousness.

Cyclic vomiting in children; and what is commonly called 'feeling liverish'.

Certain allergic conditions, such as nettle-rash, asthma and hay fever. Some of the antibodies the body uses to fight allergies are manufactured in the liver.

Gout, which is a metabolic disease of the liver.

A tendency to bruise easily, presumably because a weak liver will not produce enough prothrombin, or other clotting agents.

Weak eyesight, pain in, behind or round the eyes and black spots or zig-zags floating in front of them. The traditional Chinese belief in the relationship between eyes and liver may explain this condition.

An inability to wake fresh and alert in the morning, however early one has gone to bed, is often due to the liver (Fig. 14).

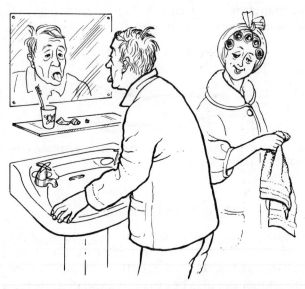

Fig. 14. Husband: 'I feel dreadful as if I had been on the tiles all night.'
   Wife: 'But you went to bed at 10 p.m. You must be livery and need a needle.'

Some weakness or disorder of the liver is commonly (though not invariably) at the root of all these troubles.

Case History. One patient of mine, a photographer, had suffered from migraine for about twenty years. The attacks would come on him once or twice a week, sometimes lasting throughout the day, so that, though he often forced himself to carry on with his work, he was equally often compelled to give up and retire to bed in a darkened room. This meant that he could never be sure of fulfilling his obligations.

When he came to me, I treated him by needling acupuncture points liver 8 and a related point, gall bladder 20 (Fig. 15). The relationship of these two points illustrates, to the acupuncturist, the known physiological interaction between the liver and the gall bladder.

I treated the patient ten times at these two points. As a result, though he still has an attack of the migraine about four times a year, he is otherwise well.

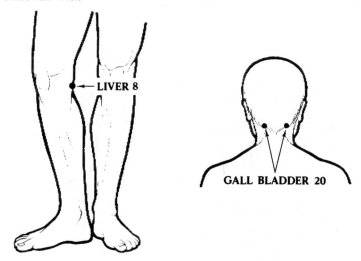

Fig. 15. These acupuncture points may be used in treating migraine.

Branches of the Main Meridian

The main meridian has various subsidiary branches supplying areas of the body adjacent to it. The dotted line in Fig. 16 shows how the branch of the heart meridian traverses the lungs, goes to the big blood vessels entering and leaving the heart, penetrates the diaphragm and connects with the small intestine. Another part of this branch travels through the throat to the eye. It is not hard to see how the main meridian's sphere of influence is enlarged by its various branches.

Case History. An elderly woman came to me some years ago complaining of her eyes, which were red, tender and sensitive to strong light. The stimulation of acupuncture point heart 3 at the elbow (see Fig. 16) cured this condition, presumably because the upper branch of the heart meridian connects with the eye.

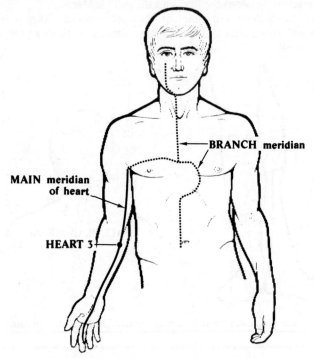

Fig. 16. The treatment of tender, red eyes, via the branch meridian.

Indirect Course of the Main Meridian

Normally the course of the main meridian is taken as the line connecting various acupuncture points along the same meridian. The liver meridian, for example, runs over the inside of the leg and over the abdomen, thus influencing diseases along its course. It also influences not only diseases of the liver itself but those related to the liver by physiology, embryology, anatomy, function etc.

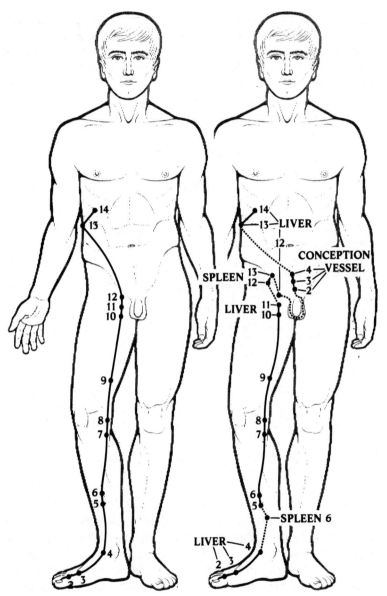

Fig. 17. Direct course of main liver meridian.

Indirect course of main liver meridian.

In reality the route taken by the liver meridian is much less direct. It changes its course by joining acupuncture points of other meridians above the ankle and in the lower abdomen, making a detour to the sex organs, which the direct course merely bypasses (Fig. 17). It can be compared to a traffic diversion on the original London to Brighton road becoming later on the main through route.

Case History. A patient had painful periods, which caused her to remain in bed two days a month. Being a pharmacist by profession, she had tried various drugs unavailingly. I needled her once a month, halfway between the periods, at liver 8 on the inside of the knee till, after six treatments, she was cured and has been free of pain for the last ten years. From an acupuncture point of view one could say the cure was affected because the indirect course of the liver meridian goes to the sex organs.

The Connecting Meridian

The connecting meridians link together the meridians of what are called coupled organs, such as the stomach and spleen, bladder and kidney or gall bladder and liver.

This takes place at the so-called connecting points, where the coupled meridians pass close to one another. The amount of tissue traversed by this part of the connecting meridian is too small to alter the symptomatology associated with the meridians position; but the importance of the connection is that it offers a means whereby stimulating the bladder for example will affect not only the bladder but also the kidney.

There is another division of the connecting meridian considerably longer than the part which goes to the coupled meridian. This division leaves the main meridian at the connecting point; then, after (as a rule) following it for some distance, finally disperses in a region not traversed by the main meridian.

Figure 18 shows how that part of the stomach connecting meridian which crosses the side of the neck and goes behind the ear is not covered by the main or any other parts of the meridian.

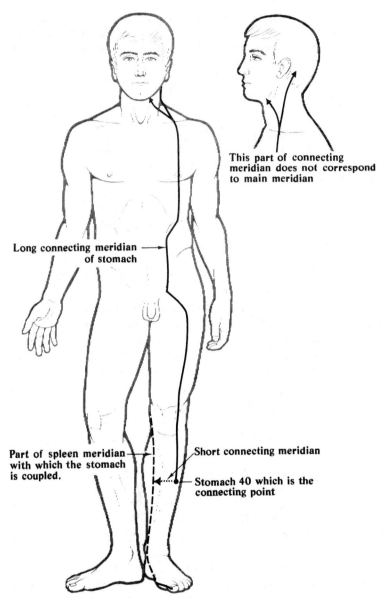

Fig. 18. The connecting meridian of the stomach may be used in treating a stiff neck.

Case History. An elderly gentleman complained of a stiffness in his neck, particularly at the sides and behind the ears, which prevented him from turning his head easily. He said it was important to him as a motorist to be able to glance rapidly from side to side, since he liked to relieve the monotony of driving by looking at pretty girls on the pavements. By treating point stomach 40 on the shin (Fig. 18) and a few local points on the neck I enabled him to recapture all his old enthusiasm.

An X-ray of his neck, however, showed rather advanced osteo-arthritis and bone can only grow again to a limited extent, so this sprightly old gentleman needed a single pep up treatment two or three times a year thereafter.

The Muscle Meridian

In all there are twelve muscle meridians. They are thought to affect chiefly muscles and joints, and have no connections with the interior of the body. Figures 19*a* and *b* show how

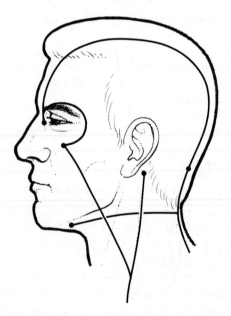

Fig. 19a. Muscle meridian of bladder.

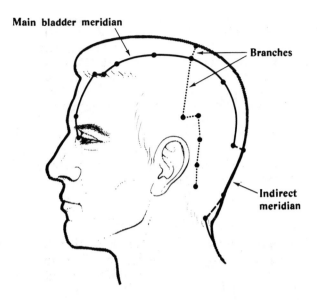

Fig. 19b. Main, indirect and branch meridians of bladder.

widely the course taken by the bladder muscle meridian in the head and neck differs from that of the main, the indirect or the branch meridian.

It will be obvious that a patient with neuralgia above and beside the eye may be treated through the bladder meridian, as this area is covered by the bladder muscle meridian.

The Divergent Meridian

Six of the twelve main meridians do not directly reach the head; but they are able to reach it indirectly by a divergent meridian which leaves the main to join the coupled meridian. This continues on into the head.

The course of the divergent meridians also differs in some respects from that of the main meridian. Figure 20 shows the course of the bladder and kidney divergent meridian; but there are five further pairs of divergent meridians.

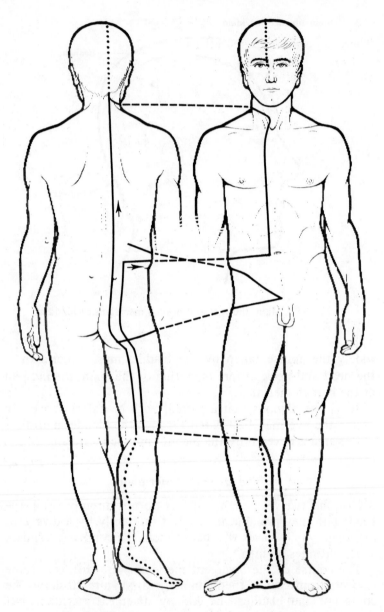

Fig. 20. Bladder and kidney divergent meridians.

The Extra Meridian

There are eight extra meridians.

Two of these, the governing vessel and vessel of conception, run along the middle of the body and have their own acupuncture points. The main effect of stimulating these acupuncture points is on organs at the same level. If for example a patient has a duodenal or stomach ulcer, it could be treated by points conception vessel 12 or governing vessel 5.5 (Fig. 21).

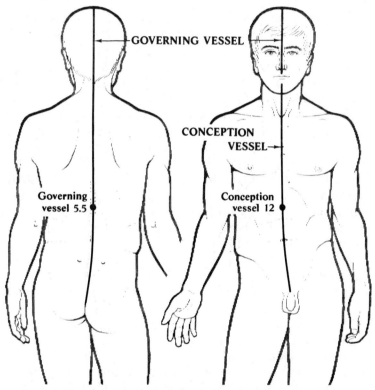

Fig. 21. The treatment of duodenal ulcer via the extra meridians.

The six other extra meridians join together certain of the main meridians and one or two points on them are supposed to activate the whole meridian.

PRACTICAL APPLICATION

The Meridian Complex

Traditionally the various types of meridians are described as being separate entities, each type having its own particular function; but, for practical purposes, I do not think the difference between the various types amounts to very much.

For example, a symptom at least partially localised over the cheek might suggest some dysfunction of the bladder muscle meridian, which unites there. If pulse diagnosis and other symptoms or signs also indicate a dysfunction of the bladder, the diagnosis is confirmed; and the disease may be treated by acupuncture points on the bladder main meridian or by points on other meridians which have an indirect effect on the bladder.

This shows that the specialised types of meridians enlarge the field of the main ones; and I myself consider it best to see them as an extension of the main meridian bearing the name of the same organ. Thus the use of an acupuncture point on the gall bladder main meridian has its field of activity extended to the connecting, muscle, divergent and branch meridians of the gall bladder. Conversely, a symptom along or near any of the above specialised meridians indicates some disturbance of the gall bladder.

Many parts of the body are not near any particular one of the twelve main meridians, but if these are taken together with all the other meridians (a total of 59), practically every part of the body is covered.

The vessel of conception and governing vessel could be counted as a special addition, for they have their own acupuncture points, thus making a total of fourteen important meridians. The other six extra meridians do not seem to fit in with the above classification. It is possible that they channel the influences of particular points, such as kidney 3, which have a large sphere of activity. Alternatively, they may act as communications between various meridians, and would therefore be classified under the meridian to which they have the greatest affinity, e.g. the girdle vessel as part of the gall bladder complex.

In many parts of the body several meridians, each belonging to a different member of the main twelve, run over the same area. Where this occurs, detection of the offending meridian entails not only noting pulse diagnosis, symptoms and signs, but also requires a knowledge of the principles of physiology and pathology. In every such instance one has to take into account all the above factors, the relation of the meridian to the diseased area being but one of many. These often contradict one another and need to be weighed in the light of clinical experience (Fig. 22).

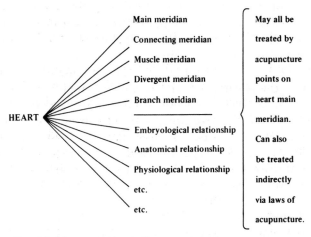

Fig. 22. The pervading influence of the important organs.

Case History. A patient whom I saw from Australia had recurrent bouts of severe abdominal pain. It started at the level of the navel, worse on the left than the right, and after two days went to the left side of the back. His stools were pale before an attack and he was constipated during the attack. He had been to hospital many times and was losing weight and sleep. Laboratory tests were suggestive of a disease of the pancreas.

The meridians which run over the part of the abdomen and back where he had pain are those of the kidney, bladder, stomach and spleen. The problem was solved by the Chinese pulse diagnosis (see

Chapter IX) which showed a dysfunction of the kidney (and the lung—though this is of secondary importance).

Ten treatments over a period of three months cured his condition. Later when he went back to Australia his wife wrote: 'He is a changed man, he has gained 1½ stone and eats and sleeps better than ever before'.

The Organ Affects the Meridian and the Meridian Affects the Organ

The meridians are, as it were, the threads linking the various phenomena observable in acupuncture both in diagnosis and treatment.

A patient may have a disease of the heart. Amongst other things, this is usually accompanied by pain down the inside of the arm roughly along the course of the heart meridian. There may also be pain going up the throat to the eye, or over the chest to the middle of the abdomen, these pains following the course of the branches of the main heart meridian or of the muscle or connecting or divergent heart meridian. If an acupuncture point on the heart meridian is stimulated in this type of case, the disease of the heart (provided it is the type of cardiac disease treatable by acupuncture) will be cured, or at least ameliorated.

These events may be reversed in a patient who has sprained or fractured his wrist in such a way as to produce a particularly tender place over the meridian of the heart. Without having had any previous cardiac symptoms, he may suddenly develop palpitations or a feeling of constriction in his chest or a difficulty in breathing after exertion. This patient, too, may be cured by the stimulation of an acupuncture point on the meridian of the heart, using the meridian either on both sides, or on the same side as the injury, or preferably only the opposite side (Fig. 23).

Thus a disease or dysfunction of the heart may cause symptoms along one or other of the meridians belonging to the heart complex; conversely, an irritation of a certain point on the heart meridian may cause cardiac symptoms or even disease. But in either case, whether originating in the heart itself or from an irritation of the heart meridian, the disease or dysfunction may be corrected by stimulating acupuncture points on the meridian of the heart.

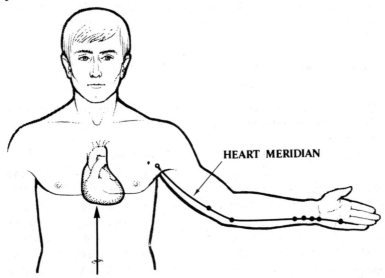

HEART MERIDIAN

Fig. 23. A disease of the heart may weaken structures along the course of the heart meridian, so that it is easier to have a sprain there, have rheumatism, neuritis etc.

A sprain, broken bone or anything else along the course of the heart meridian may cause heart symptoms such as palpitations, breathlessness or a feeling of pressure on the chest.

This illustrates one of the special advantages of acupuncture, since diagnosis and treatment can be in such close alliance as to be practically the same thing. If, that is, one is confident of the diagnosis, one more or less automatically knows the treatment; if, on the other hand, one is unsure of the diagnosis and tries out some particular treatment which proves successful, the diagnosis as automatically follows.

The Meridians and Cellular Pathology

Western medicine is based on the system of cellular pathology, as first expounded by Virchow. This distinguishes as minutely as possible the type of the diseased tissue (whether muscle, bone, blood-vessel, nerve etc), which type of cell in that tissue is diseased and, recently, even the intra-cellular changes that take place in the diseased cell.

In acupuncture, the reverse of these ideas often seem to apply. An insect bite on the elbow, for instance, is best treated in acupuncture by stimulating the meridian which runs over that part. If, for example, the bite were in the region of the lateral bony protuberance at the elbow, the large intestine meridian (preferably on the opposite side) would be treated. If, instead of an insect bite on the elbow, the patient suffered from muscular rheumatism, a painful wound, early arthritis, tennis elbow, a localised skin disease, or any other disease involving the cellular elements in that region of the body, the treatment would be exactly the same—the stimulation of the large intestine meridian on the opposite side.

From this it may be seen that the cellular pathology does not necessarily dictate any difference in treatment by acupuncture.

It would therefore seem that the meridians are the dominant factor in the various regions of the body and that they control it chiefly in a regional way, irrespective of what type of tissue or cell may be present (Fig. 24). In addition to

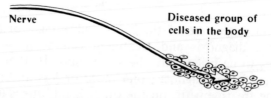

Fig. 24. The above nerve goes to a certain area of the body. It is still the same nerve, whatever the disease, and hence it is this nerve (or meridian) which has to be stimulated.

this, they have an effect on the whole body, which appears to operate through the mediation of the internal organs with which the meridians are connected.

A knowledge of microscopic anatomy and cellular pathology is nevertheless important in acupuncture in a more general way, in helping to decide which disease can or cannot be treated. A duodenal ulcer, for instance, may be treated successfully, as the cells lining the duodenum are of a type which regenerate easily. Disease of the central nervous system, however, can be treated only to a limited extent, for the neurones of the brain and spinal cord do not appreciably regenerate.

Case History. An accountant of 29 had a stomach ulcer for 15 years. It had twice perforated. Because of the danger of further perforations he had two thirds of his stomach removed at operation when he was 22. (His father and brother had also had their stomachs excised.) Despite this he continued to have heartburn nearly every day, frequently vomiting a third of a pint of acid fluid half an hour before meals, and also suddenly within seconds he would sometimes lose his appetite.

After twelve treatments he was practically symptom free. In this case although acupuncture could, of course, not make the missing two thirds of the stomach grow again, what was left was so fortified as to take over the function of the missing part. As the cure could not be complete he needed a pep up treatment every quarter year.

V

THE FIVE ELEMENTS

'The five elements, wood, fire, earth, metal, water, encompass all the phenomena of nature. It is a symbolism that applies itself equally to man'.

(Su Wen)

Certain things in the practice of acupuncture can be better understood in the light of the Chinese belief that five elements comprise the world and that to one, or more than one, of these elements everything on earth essentially belongs.

This recalls to mind the four elements, earth, water, air, and fire, which were a familiar part of Western practice till comparatively recent times; nor is it difficult to see that the nature of everything in the world places it in one or several of these categories. For example, a brick belongs to the element earth; a glass of wine to the elements earth (glass) and water (wine); a barrage balloon to the elements earth (the balloon) and air (helium); a coal fire to earth (coal), air (carbon dioxide and other gases) and fire. ·

These four elements are common to both the European and the Chinese systems (though in the latter the equivalent of Air is Metal). The fifth element is known only to the Chinese and to certain other civilisations whose roots extend to prehistoric times. It is called 'wood'.

The name alludes to the mysterious and much debated element of 'life'. The first four elements are concerned with the physical life we can apprehend with our five senses, and they can therefore only describe the inanimate world or, at best, the inanimate in the animate. The fifth element seeks to describe the animate itself, the living plant, whose ligneous skeleton is its most permanent structure.

The element wood might appear to have been added to the other four merely as a means of explaining away the phenomenon of life. But in the Chinese system, wood is the original element from which the other four were evolved; in the beginning was life (wood), the first of the elements; from it afterwards developed matter (the remaining four).

It is interesting to note certain correlations with the West. In China the life (wood) element was thought to live in the organ known as the liver; and the idea, though we in the West no longer believe in it, forms part of the structure of our language. Liver—life; Leber—Leben. The words have the same stem in both English and German. It is mainly in the liver that those metabolic processes take place which make life possible; and to the liver, at least in this connection, the other organs are subsidiary. The kidney excretes the products of metabolism; the lungs take in oxygen as fuel for the

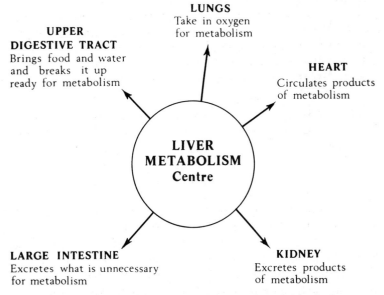

LUNGS
Take in oxygen
for metabolism

**UPPER
DIGESTIVE TRACT**
Brings food and water
and breaks it up
ready for metabolism

HEART
Circulates products
of metabolism

**LIVER
METABOLISM
Centre**

LARGE INTESTINE
Excretes what is unnecessary
for metabolism

KIDNEY
Excretes products
of metabolism

Fig. 25. The liver is the most important organ in the body.

metabolic process; the heart circulates the products of the liver (Fig. 25). The viability and regenerative power of the liver exceed that of all other organs whether in the living body or in tissue culture.

To the Western world this idea of a fifth element concerned with 'life' itself has about it a flavour of the mysterious or esoteric; but in reading ancient Chinese literature on the element wood, one is immediately struck by the matter-of-fact tone in which it is described. It is precisely the same tone as that used in describing any other obvious everyday event, no more and no less ordinary than the thousand events man takes for granted merely because they are familiar. This down-to-earth attitude, together with certain other indications, suggests that these ancient races were endowed with a faculty for the perception of forces which the civilised man of today is no longer able to appreciate. It is probably one reason why the element wood was not recognised by relatively more modern western civilisations.

The five elements, then, are:

> Wood
> Fire
> Earth
> Metal (Air, in the western tradition)
> Water

The interplay of these five primeval forces, linked in an unvarying pattern one to another, brought into being the macrocosm, which is mirrored by the 'little world' of man. The rhythm of this eternal dance of the elements is illustrated in Fig. 26, the outer lines representing the creative and the inner ones the destructive forces.

Wood will burn to create a *Fire*; which when it has finished burning, leaves behind the ashes, *Earth*; from which may be mined the *Metals*; which, if heated, become molten like *Water*; which is necessary for the growth of plants and *Wood*. This is the creative cycle.

Wood destroys *Earth*, i.e. plants can crack rocks and break up the soil. *Earth* destroys *Water*, i.e. a jug with its earthenware sides prevents water from following its natural law of spreading out. *Water* destroys *Fire*, i.e. water, poured over a fire, will extinguish it. *Fire* destroys *Metal*, i.e. by melting. *Metal* destroys *Wood*, i.e. by cutting.

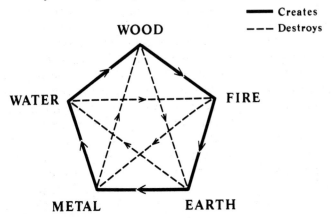

Fig. 26. The five elements. One of the theoretical bases of Chinese medicine and philosophy.

In medicine the law of the five elements is applied as follows:

Yin	*Yang*
Wood is equivalent to the Liver	and Gall Bladder
Fire is equivalent to the Heart	and Small Intestine
Earth is equivalent to the Spleen	and Stomach·
Metal is equivalent to the Lung	and Large Intestine
Water is equivalent to the Kidney	and Bladder
Fire is equivalent to the Pericardium	and Triple Warmer

It should be understood that these terms 'Wood', 'Fire', etc were not used by the Chinese in the actual restrictive sense of the physical wood, fire etc., but rather as implying an archetypal idea, in the sense in which it is used by the psychologist Jung, himself a profound student of Chinese philosophy. For example, the *idea* of the genus house is opposed to the idea of an *actual* house. Before a man can build a house he must have conceived the idea of 'house', whether a bungalow, a skyscraper, a family home for the miner or an olde Tudor cottage for the retired business man. The generic idea of 'house' is primary and covers a vast number of possibilities; an actual house built of bricks and mortar etc. is only secondary to the general idea comprising all houses.

Thus what I have expressed above as '*Metal* destroys *Wood*', i.e. wood may be cut by a metal saw, is the expression in material terms of what is essentially an idea, though it may manifest itself in various physical guises such as wood or the liver.

In the actual practice of acupuncture this theory of the five elements dictates that when the liver (wood) is tonified,

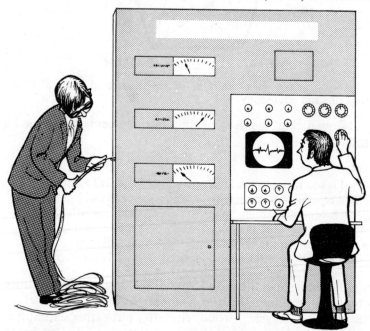

Fig. 27. A computer has been invented to calculate all the direct and indirect effects of a needle prick via the many laws of acupuncture. Symptoms fed in can be analysed and some guidance given as to treatment. An experienced doctor practising acupuncture can perform diagnosis and assess the correct treatment, without a computer.

the heart (fire) will automatically be also tonified, while the spleen (earth) is sedated; or, if the kidney (water) is sedated, the liver (wood) will automatically be sedated too and the heart (fire) tonified.

This relationship of the internal organs may sound to certain doctors like sheer nonsense. But I know from my own experience that, when studying acupuncture, I did not always take full account of the various aspects of the law of the five elements. It needs something like a mathematical calculation if, for a single needle prick, one has to consider all the possible repercussions of the laws of 'mother-son', 'husband-wife', deep and superficial circulations of energy, 'midday-midnight' etc., which are mentioned later in this book. Every now and then I obtained unexpected results from pulse diagnosis of my patients' symptoms, and it was only when I began to take into account the rules of the law of five elements as well as all the other laws that it became possible to explain these results (Fig. 27).

Case History. Recently I saw a young trendy gentleman, who had to buy several new suits a year as his excessive perspiration caused them to rot and stain. He perspired summer and winter and had to sponge his suit every day to prevent salt rings forming.

Theoretically this condition could be due to an underactivity of the skin for the Chinese say that the pores open and close properly only when the skin is healthy—and the skin as will be seen later in this chapter is activated by the lungs. The sweating could also be due to: the kidneys not excreting enough water; the heart being weak and causing a sweat as in fainting; a dysfunction of the liver or spleen which may cause water retention.

As shown above, organs belonging to any of the five elements may be at fault to produce the same symptoms of excessive sweating. A knowledge of the subject though should show without undue difficulty which is the culprit—in this young man's case the lung and kidney.

Certain of these relationships are obvious in the practice of ordinary medicine, i.e., tonification of the kidney (water) will produce by its increased excretion of water and solids a tonification (decongestion) of the liver (wood) and also a sedation of the heart (fire) which no longer has to force too much fluid through the body. A fuller explanation, however, will require much more research from the side of ordinary science.

This general classification of the five elements is worked out in greater detail for those acupuncture points that lie between the fingertips and the elbow and between the tips of the toes and the knees, a series of points whereby it is possible to treat nearly any disease wherever it may appear on the body, without having recourse to any other acupuncture points (Fig. 28 and 29).

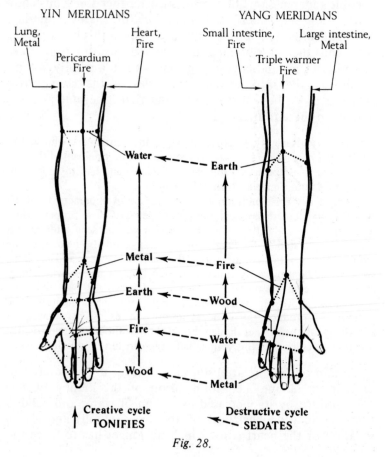

YIN MERIDIANS   YANG MERIDIANS

Lung, Metal   Heart, Fire   Small intestine, Fire   Large intestine, Metal

Pericardium Fire   Triple warmer Fire

Water ← ─ ─ ─ Earth

Metal ← ─ ─ ─ Fire

Earth ← ─ ─ ─ Wood

Fire ← ─ ─ ─ Water

Wood ← ─ ─ ─ Metal

Creative cycle
TONIFIES

Destructive cycle
SEDATES

Fig. 28.

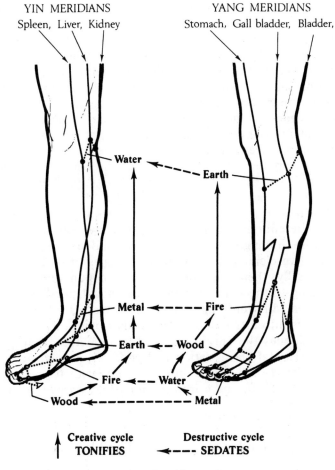

Fig. 29.

It will be noted that the direction of movement is centripetal, from the finger or toe tips inwards in accordance with the creative cycle, i.e., from the finger tip, anterior surface, wood, fire, earth, etc. Equivalent positions on the anterior and posterior surfaces are, by the law of five elements, antagonistic to one another. i.e., at the finger tip metal and wood are antagonistic in such a manner that the external surface (metal) is the destructive agent. Thus both the creative and the destructive cycles are centripetal, moving from without inwards, i.e., from the tips of fingers or toes to the elbow or knee (creative cycle); or from the posterior surface, which is embryologically an external surface, to the anterior surface, which is embryologically a more internal surface (destructive cycle).

The arrangement of the elements on the anterior surface of the arm is the same as that on the medial (embryologically anterior) surface of the leg. Similarly, the arrangement of the elements on the posterior surface of the arm is the same as the arrangement of those on the lateral (embryologically posterior) surface of the leg.

It will also be noted that the five element rule is applied in two different senses. The drawings show that each of the vertically running meridians in the arm and leg belongs to one of the five elements; while at right angles to these, running horizontally, there are groups of three acupuncture points all belonging to the same element, even though they are placed on three different meridians. The classification of the meridians into elements I have found of practical value since, if one applies the ensuing laws of acupuncture, they work. The horizontal classification is, I consider, largely incorrect.

The heart and small intestine are said to belong to 'princely fire', the pericardium and triple warmer to 'ministerial fire'.

Extension of the Law of Five Elements

From one point of view the whole universe was considered in ancient China to be divisible into five groups. From other points of view it was divisible into two groups, the Yang and the Yin (male-female; hot-cold; light-dark; positive-negative); into twelve groups—the basic twelve organs and meridians; or again into ten groups—the basic Tsang (solid) and Fu (hollow) organs, their ten celestial stems, etc.

This numerical division of the universe is foreign to our way of thinking and may seem arbitrary, but a little reflection should make its plausibility evident. There are statements of the same truth in different terms:

In terms of electricity the world is divided into two—those objects that have predominantly a positive charge and those that have predominantly a negative charge. On a fine day, for example, the atmospheric electricity is mainly positive, while on a cloudy day it is negative. The inside of a single human cell is negative, the surface positive—so long as the cell is alive. All chemical elements have their so-called electro-chemical potential according to their ratio of positive and negative charges, etc.

In terms of chemical elements the world is divided into ninety-two natural elements such as copper (No. 29), carbon (No. 6), calcium (No. 20), oxygen (No. 8), tin (No. 5), uranium (No. 92). Everything material that exists contains various proportions of several of these elements.

In terms of general science everything is divisible into three — animal, vegetable and mineral.

Likewise, in terms of the law of the five elements everything is divisible in fives, of which a partial chart is given on p. 50.

I myself have not been able to verify all the factors mentioned in the chart overleaf, and I have my doubts about the correctness of a few of them, but that the majority are correct I have no doubt as I use them in diagnosis and treatment with success.

It is well known, for example, that someone who has a liver (wood) weakness is more sensitive than the average to an East (wood) wind (wood), that his nails (wood) may be blemished and that he may have foggy vision with black spots (wood). That the person who feels cold (water) in his bones (water) is found by the pulse diagnosis to have a weakness of the kidneys (water). That the person who talks (fire) incessantly with a high colour (fire) has an overactivity of the heart (fire). That the frightened (water) child who does not want to sleep in the dark and wets (water) his bed has a weakness of the kidney (water). That the diabetic (earth) who eats too much sugar (earth) will propably end up with a

Element	Wood	Fire	Earth	Metal	Water
Yin organ	Liver	Heart	Spleen	Lungs	Kidney
Yang organ	Gall bladder	Small intestine	Stomach	Large intestine	Bladder
Sense commanded	Slight	Words	Taste	Smell	Hearing
Nourishes the	Muscles	Blood vessels	Fat	Skin	Bones
Expands into the	Nails	Colour	Lips	Body hair	Hair on head
Liquid emitted	Tears	Sweat	Saliva	Mucus	Urine
Bodily smell	Rancid	Scorched	Fragrant	Fleshy	Putrid
Associated temperament	Depressed	Emotions up & down	Obsession	Anguish	Fear
	Anger	Joy	Sympathy	Grief	
Flavour	*Sour	Bitter	Sweet	Hot	Salt
Sound	Shout	Laugh	Sing	Weep	Groan
Dangerous type of weather	Wind	Heat	Humidity	Dryness	Cold
Season	Spring	Summer	Mid-summer	Autumn	Winter
Colour	Green	Red	Yellow	White	Black
Direction	East	South	Centre	West	North
Beneficial cereal	Wheat	Millet	Rye	Rice	Beans
Beneficial meat	Chicken	Mutton	Beef	Horse	Pork
Musical note	chio	chih	kung	shang	yu

* Sour like vinegar, bitter like bitter melon, sweet like sugar, hot like ginger, salt like table salt.

diabetic (earth) coma, and that the renal (water) hypertensive who eats too much salt (water) may finish prematurely in the grave.

Indirect effects, though more rarely found, must not be forgotten. Foggy vision (wood) is normally due to an under-activity of the liver (wood), but occasionally to an under-active kidney (water) [which is the 'mother'* by the law of five elements].

This system may also be used therapeutically:

In psychology (Fig. 30) a person with an endogenous depression (wood) may be cured by treating the liver (wood). Someone who weeps (metal) a lot may after the destructive cycle of the five elements be told to laugh (fire) more, which naturally would put a stop to the weepiness. If that is not enough, the heart (fire) itself may be stimulated either by

* See later chapters.

acupuncture or by giving the correct cardiac (fire) tonic or eating bitter (fire) food—though as a rule the more powerful stimulus of acupuncture is most effective.

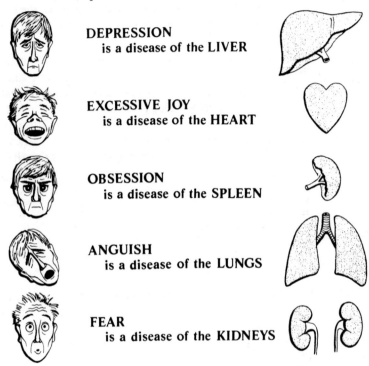

DEPRESSION
is a disease of the LIVER

EXCESSIVE JOY
is a disease of the HEART

OBSESSION
is a disease of the SPLEEN

ANGUISH
is a disease of the LUNGS

FEAR
is a disease of the KIDNEYS

Fig. 30. Acupuncture and psychology.

Case history. I once saw a patient who was unable to stop talking (words-fire). The pulse diagnosis revealed an overactivity of the pulse of the heart (fire) and I therefore stimulated acupuncture point heart 7. Within a few minutes of the needle being in place the constant chatter stopped and the patient spoke normally for about a day when the incessant flow of words started again. A repetition of similar treatment brought about a cure.

Case History. A patient had nails (wood) which kept cracking and were thin and brittle with longitudinal ridges (calcium had been tried to no avail). Her eyes (wood) watered very easily, especially in the wind (wood). Her body had a slightly rancid (wood) smell and she easily became angry (wood) when she would shout (wood) a lot. The pulse diagnosis revealed an underactivity of the liver (wood). As the 'mother'* of wood is water, point liver 8 (the water point) on the liver meridian was used. This or similar treatment was repeated to effect a cure.

It is interesting to note that the improvement started within two weeks of initiating treatment. Yet a nail takes some four months to grow up from its base, which suggests that the theory of the physiology of nails needs a little revision. This observation has been made repeatedly with various patients: the time response may vary, but is always faster than would be expected from the speed of growth of the nail.

* See later chapters

VI

THE ENERGY OF LIFE-Qi

The ancient Chinese made no precise distinction between arteries, veins, lymphatics, nerves, tendons or meridians. They were concerned rather with a system of Forces in the body, those forces which enable a man to move, breathe, digest his food and think. As in other so-called primitive systems of medicine, like the Egyptian or the Aztec, the anatomical structures which make these physiological processes possible were not described in detail. They concentrated instead on this elaborate system of forces, whose interplay regulated all the functions of the body.

In Western medicine we have an intricate knowledge of anatomy, microscope anatomy, the chemistry and biochemistry of the body but little knowledge of what actually makes it 'tick'. It was this energy at the roots of all life which was the primary interest of the ancient Chinese.

Life Energy (Qi)

Qi (life energy) is one of the fundamental concepts of Chinese thought. The manifestation of any invisible force, whether it be the growth of a plant, the movement of an arm or the deafening thunder of a storm, is called Qi: though, as we shall see, there are many varieties of it, each with its own specific function. In Hindu terminology the nearest equivalent to Qi is 'Prana'; in Theosopy and Anthroposophy it is called the 'Ether' or 'Etheric Body' (Fig. 31).

Qi in the human body is called True Qi and is created by breathing and eating. The Qi inhaled from the air is extracted by the lungs, the Qi in food and water by the stomach and its associated organ the spleen.

Fig. 31. The blank space in the box represents Qi: it cannot be weighed or measured, for according to the ancient Chinese it is non-material. Its effect, though, can be seen in the growth of a plant, the power of thought, the energy that activates any process. Much of this (though by no means all) can be explained in a different way via the materialistic laws of science. Insofar as it applies to acupuncture the flow of Qi along meridians, would in modern medicine be described as an electrical impulse (depolarisation) travelling along a nerve.

'True Qi is a combination of what is received from the heavens and the Qi of water and food. It permeates the whole body.'

(Ling Shu, cilie zhenxie pian)

Western medicine would explain death from asphyxiation as due to lack of air and death from starvation or dehydration to lack of food or water. The ancient Chinese neither ignored nor denied these obvious physical facts but they did not consider them to be the complete explanation. That must include the lack of the vital energy of life. The inability of the body to extract Qi from air, food and water is just as much a cause of death as its deprivation of them.

In these particular instances it is clear that the physical and metaphysical phenomena, deriving from the same source, cannot readily be distinguished. In others the difference can be more easily observed.

'*True Qi is the original Qi. Qi from Heaven is received through the nose and controlled by the wind-pipe; Qi from food and water enters the stomach and is controlled by the gullet. That which nourishes the unborn is the Qi of former heaven (pre-natal); that which fills the born is called the Qi of the latter heaven (post-natal).*'

(Zhangshi leijing)

Qi is universal:

'*The root of the way of life (Dao or Tao), of birth and change is Qi; the myriad things of heaven and earth all obey this law. Thus Qi in periphery envelops heaven and earth, Qi in the interior activates them. The source wherefrom the sun, moon and stars derive their light, the thunder, rain, wind and cloud their being, the four seasons and the myriad things their birth, growth, gathering and storing: all this is brought about by Qi. Man's possession of life is completely dependent upon this Qi.*'

(Zhangshi leijing)

Before a mother can conceive and the foetus develop, her body, according to the Chinese, must be in harmony. The two extra meridians called the vessel of conception and the penetrating vessel should be active and the umbilical cord properly functioning. Only then can the Qi of former heaven be adequately received by the mother. After birth the Qi of former heaven is cut off as the baby begins to take in from the air it breathes and from the digestion of food and water the Qi of latter heaven.

Qi activates all the processes of the body, '*the unceasing circulation of the blood, the dissemination of fluid in skin and flesh, joints and bone-hollows, the lubrication of the digestive tract, sweating, urination etc.*' In Chinese treatises on acupuncture the effect of pricking the skin with a needle is called 'obtaining Qi'; if the needle fails to obtain Qi (which is often indicated by various signs and symptoms) the acupuncture treatment will be ineffective.

'Thus one is able to smell only if Lung Qi penetrates to the nose; one can distinguish the five colours only if Liver Qi penetrates to the eyes; one can taste only if Heart Qi penetrates to the tongue; one can know whether one likes or dislikes food only if Spleen Qi penetrates to the mouth.'

'The capabilities of the seven holes (eyes, ears, nose and mouth) depend upon the penetration of the Qi from the five solid organs' (as mentioned in the preceding paragraph).

(Zhongyixue gailun)

'That which was from the beginning in heaven is Qi; on earth it becomes visible as form; Qi and form interact, giving birth to the myriad things.'

(Su Wen, Ch. 66)

The cycle of changes which results from the interaction of Qi and form is what the Chinese meant when they described the 'transformation of air, food and water into Qi, blood and other substances'. This is the transformation at work in the rhythms of growth and decay, in the changes from the flower to the fruit or the child to the old man.

The meridians are the tracks along which travel many of the impulses mentioned above—or, as the Chinese put it, *'the meridians are the paths of the transforming action of Qi in the solid and hollow organs'* (Yijiang jingyi).

The word Qi in Chinese has, besides 'Life Energy', the further meaning of 'Air'. Only over the last hundred years, since it became possible to weigh air by creating a true vacuum, has it been defined as physical. To the Chinese air was non-material and could therefore only be a vehicle for the forces of energy. Thus they often use the phrase 'bad Qi' for what we, more prosaically, would call a bad smell. This double meaning of air and energy may be an explanation of the breathing exercises in Indian Yoga; the Chinese use a similar system to obtain Qi.

Other Varieties of Qi

Qi as such is the primeval force that permeates everything. There are, however, specialised varieties of it with different functions in the body, much as water has a different function from ingested food.

Qi in Relation to Acupuncture

To the ancients the cornerstone of the theory of acupuncture, the concept whereby they explained its effects and action, was Qi, the energy of life. Nowadays acupuncture can be explained by a wave of electrical depolarisation that travels along nerves, an idea which is really not so very different from that held by the ancient Chinese and relatively easy to be correlated with it.

The Chinese thought of Qi as flowing along the meridians, much as water flows along a river-bed or a nervous impulse along a nerve. The meridians and their smaller and smallest branches irrigated like a river the whole country (the human body). If a disease arose in the body it affected these rivers of life, so that either no water flowed at all (lack of Qi) or the river was blocked with excessive water and flooding above the block (swelling, and congestion of Qi) and insufficient water below the block (atrophy, lack of Qi). It was thought that in some way the acupuncture needle removed the block, either directly or by increasing the force of the stream.

The twelve main meridians run round the body thrice. The cycle (Fig. 32 to 34) starts with the lung (1) meridian on the front of the chest, which goes to the hand; then the large intestine (2) meridian, which goes from the hand to the face; then the stomach (3) meridian, which goes from the head down to the foot; then the spleen (4) meridian, which goes from the foot back to the chest near the origin of the lung meridian. This complete cycle of the body is then repeated for the meridians of heart (5), small intestine (6), bladder (7), kidney (8); and then again repeated for the third and final time by the meridians of pericardium (9), triple warmer (10), gall bladder (11), liver (12). It is this continuous flow of Qi which carries the pulse of life.

Case History. A schoolboy had little energy. He did not have enough energy to listen to his teacher, do his homework, or play games. Evenings and weekends he sat around doing nothing. He was rather flat chested. I treated his lungs on several occasions, giving him more zest in life and enabling him to move up in his form.

The traditional Chinese would have said that the boy had insufficient Qi in his lungs.

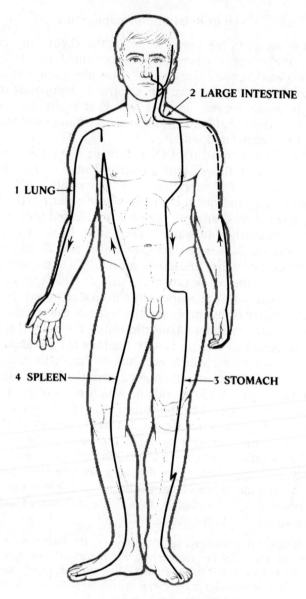

Fig. 32. The course of the meridians 1 to 4.

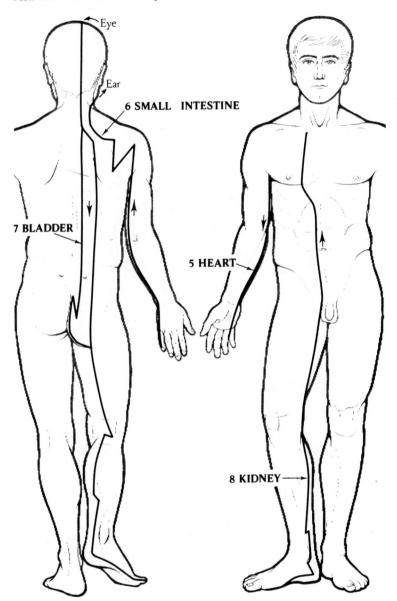

Fig. 33. The course of the meridians 5 to 8.

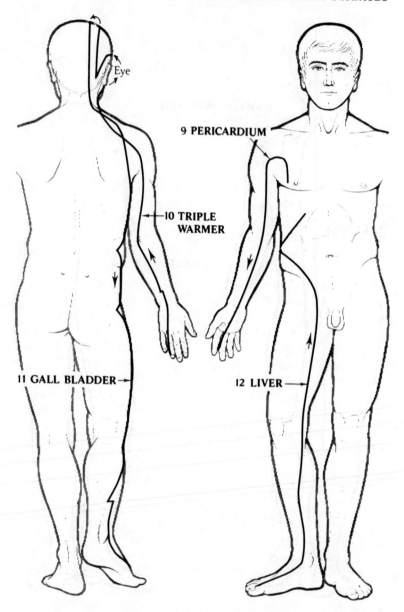

Fig. 34. The course of the meridians 9 to 12.

VII

THE LIVING INTERDEPENDENT DYNAMISM OF THE BODY

The Chinese saw the body as an organism so delicately balanced that whatever affected one part of it would have repercussions on others: a concept sadly lacking in ordinary Western medicine today. For the average doctor tends to think of the various parts of the body as relatively isolated and may even become so much a specialist in one small area as to forget that occasionally a headache may be caused by something wrong with the foot. The Chinese, though, however static their civilisation remained, had in medicine the opposite, namely a dynamic view of the body as a living unity, where every piece is so interlocked that the dislodgement of one will have an effect on some or all of the others.

This process whereby organs affect one another is not just an arbitrary process occurring haphazardly; it follows laws not unlike the laws of physics, except that the paths it takes are not nearly so strict. One must thank the genius of the Chinese for having discovered these biological laws, while the modern Western scientist has discovered the inert laws of today's science.

The Midday-Midnight Law

The Chinese consider that each of the twelve important organ-meridian-function complexes has a period of two hours during which its activity is maximal, as shown in Fig. 35. The liver for example has its maximal activity from 1 a.m. to 3 a.m., together with all the various liver meridians and any physiological, embryological or anatomical entities which are grouped under the liver, such as the liver types of migraine and presumably also the production of bile by the liver.

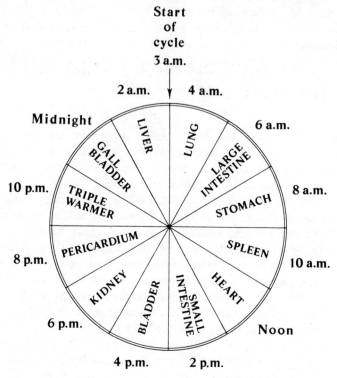

Fig. 35. Times of maximum energy.

This law may be used in diagnosis. A patient may have colicky pains which are worst at midnight (Fig. 36); and this, as reference to the diagram will show, is the period of maximal activity of the gall bladder or the period of minimal activity of the heart. Other things being equal, the pain is then most likely to be due to the gall bladder but could possibly also be due to the heart in its period of minimal activity.

This method of diagnosis, using the time of onset of symptoms, can easily be misleading. It is, however, one of the many variable factors which the astute physician can weigh up in coming to his diagnosis. Indirect effects may also occur, following the law of the five elements: the over-active gall bladder at midnight, belonging to the element wood, may itself remain symptomless, but instead influence the stomach belonging to the element earth. In this case the patient would get stomach symptoms at midnight instead of gall bladder symptoms as might be expected from a simple application of the law midday-midnight.

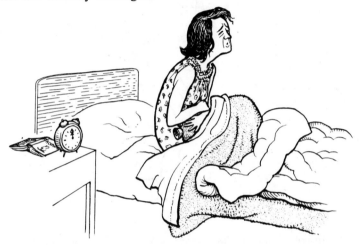

Fig. 36. Reader of this book wakes up with belly ache at midnight.
'The book on acupuncture says the gall bladder is probably wrong.

But it could be the heart as organs act on one another.
    or it could be the stomach as organs act on one another.
    or it could be the   ?   as organs act on one another.
    or it could be the   ?   as organs act on one another.
Maybe I had better leave it to the expert.'

Sometimes organs affect one another according to the midday-midnight law. Colitis is a disease in which the lining of the large intestine is inflamed, leading to diarrhoea and other intestinal symptoms. This disease may sometimes be helped by directly treating the large intestine, which has its time of maximal activity at 6 a.m., but more often treatment of the kidney, whose maximal activity is at 6 p.m., in accordance with the midday-midnight law gives better results.

At other times colitis is more effectively treated via the liver, which is outside the scope of the midday-midnight law, the colitis being merely one of several symptoms of imperfect liver function (Fig. 37).

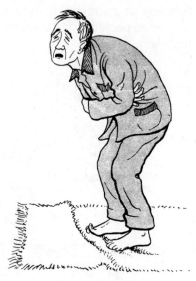

Fig. 37. In colitis one may have severe cramps in the tummy. It may be cured:

> Directly, by treating the large intestine.
> Indirectly, via the law midday-midnight by treating the kidney.
> Via the liver when it is a symptom of liver disease.
> Or by locally acting acupuncture points.

An interesting application of the law midday-midnight is the mimicry of heart (maximal activity 12 noon) and the gall bladder (maximal activity midnight) symptoms. Pain in the heart due to angina pectoris may be felt in the upper abdomen or gall bladder area, causing many people who have a heart attack to think they have indigestion.The reverse is seen in patients with an attack of acute inflammation of the gall bladder, in whom the electrocardiogram (electrical heart test) would suggest a disease of the heart.

The Mother-Son Law

'If a meridian is empty, tonify its mother. If it is full, disperse the child'.

(Zhengiu Yixue)

This quotation is normally taken to refer to the circulation of Qi through the twelve meridians, as in the circular diagram (Fig. 35). In this case, if the lung meridian is empty one should tonify its mother, the liver; if the lung is full one should disperse its child, the large intestine.

The mother-son law can occasionally apply to the law of five elements, as in the pentangular diagram (Fig. 38). In this

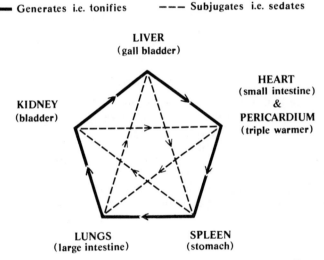

Fig. 38. Interrelationship of the five elements used in treating disease.

case, if the lung meridian is empty one should tonify its mother, the spleen; if the lung is full one should disperse its child, the kidney.

In each of the above examples (via the twelve meridians or the five elements) there are thus two alternative routes, an illustration of the variability possible in biological systems.

Case History. An 18-year-old girl suffering from acne became shy and introspective because she thought it destroyed her looks. Chinese pulse diagnosis showed a dysfunction of the liver and lung, so the liver was tonified at acupuncture point liver 14 (Fig. 39). This corrected the

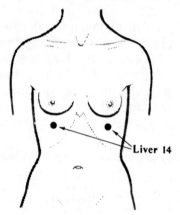

Fig. 39. One method of treating acne.

pulse of both liver and lung (as the lung follows the liver in the flow of Qi through the meridians). The result was a considerable improvement, though not a complete cure, of the acne and a corresponding improvement in the patient's attitude to life.

As the theoretical explanation shows, in different circumstances the acne could have been cured by direct treatment of the lung or, in yet other circumstances, by treating the spleen.

VIII

THE PRINCIPLE OF OPPOSITES

The Chinese believed that in the beginning the world was a formless, indivisible whole. There was no distinction between heaven and hell, fire and water, day and night; there was neither birth nor death, growth nor decay; all imaginable things were merged together without definition in an unchanging unity. Had man existed, he would have remained forever incapable of evolution, a static and perfect image.

For life to be possible as we know it, with all its richness and variety, its infinite potentialities for good and ill, this world had to be split in two. The Unity had to become a duality; and from this duality arose the idea of the complementary opposites, the negative and the positive, which the Chinese called the Yin and the Yang. These two principles are at the very root of the Chinese way of life; they pervade all their art, literature and philosophy and are therefore also embodied in their theories of traditional medicine.

These principles are, of course, up to a point accepted in the West. We too divide every phenomenon into its two contrary components. Male and female, hard and soft, good and bad, positive and negative electrical charges, laevorotary and dextrorotary chemical compounds—all these are 'opposites'. It is indeed a fact that nothing can happen in the physical world unaccompanied by positive or negative electrical changes. If a man moves his hand or a raindrop falls or a child rolls a marble across the floor, such changes will affect the balance of positive and negative charges in each of these instances. But in Europe we have not formulated this polarity as a universal law as have the Chinese, to whom the perpetual interplay of the Yin and the Yang is the very keystone of their thinking. It is the law operating throughout all existence that the states of Yin and Yang must succeed one another, so that, in a Yin condition, the corresponding Yang state can be precisely foretold. The practical application of this law to acupuncture can be illustrated thus:

	Yang	*Yin*
In the natural world:	Day	Night
	Clear day	Cloudy day
	Spring/Summer	Autumn/Winter
	East/South	West/North
	Upper	Lower
	Exterior	Interior
	Hot	Cold
	Fire	Water
	Light	Dark
	Sun	Moon
In the body:	Surfaces of body	Interior of body
	Spine/Back	Chest/abdomen
	Male	Female
	Clear or clean body fluid	Cloudy or dirty body fluid
	Energy (Qi)	Blood
	Wei	Ying
In disease:	Acute/virulent	Chronic/non-active
	Powerful/ flourishing	Weak/decaying
	Patient feels hot or hot to touch or has temperature	Patient feels cold or cold to touch or has under-temperatu
	Dry	Moist
	Advancing	Retiring
	Hasty	Lingering

The twelve basic organs and meridians are similarly divided into the Yin solid (Zang) organs, which 'store but do not transmit' and the Yang hollow (Fu) organs, 'which transform but do not retain':

Yin	Yang
Liver	Gall bladder
Heart	Small intestine
Spleen (Pancreas)	Stomach
Lung	Large intestine
Kidney	Bladder
Pericardium	Triple warmer

The qualities of Yin and Yang are relative, not absolute. For example, the surface of the body is Yang, the interior Yin; but this relation also remains constant within the body, for the surface of every internal organ is always Yang and its interior always Yin, down to the individual cells that compose it. Similarly, a gas is Yang, a solid Yin; but among the gases the more rarified are Yang, the denser are Yin. Life and death belong to Yang, growth and storage to Yin, so that 'if only Yang exists, there will be no birth: if only Yin exists, there will be no growth'. The life of every organism depends upon the correct balance of its various components.

'Yin and Yang are the Tao of heaven and earth (the basic law of opposition and unity in the natural world), the fundamental principle of the myriad things (all things can only obey this law and cannot transgress it), the originators (literally parents) of change in all things is according to this law), the beginning of birth and death (the birth and creation, death and destruction of all things begins with this law), the storehouse of Shen Ming (the location of all that is mysterious in the natural world). The treatment of disease must be sought for in this basic law (man is one of the living things of nature), so the curing of disease must be sought for in this basic law.'

(Su Wen, Ch. 5)

Since everything in life can be classified according to its Yin and Yang components (see also Fig. 40), it is said:

'Now the Yin/Yang has a name but not form. Thus it can be extended from one to ten, from ten to a hundred, from a hundred to a thousand, from a thousand to ten thousand (i.e., it can embrace all things).'

(Ling Shu, yingang xi riyue pian)

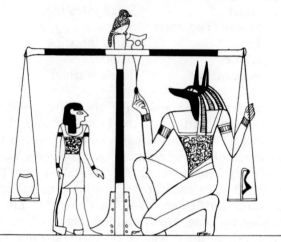

Fig. 40. Is the heart (in the jar) or the feather heavier—an aspect of Yin and Yang in ancient Egypt. After the Book of the Dead, British Museum.

From the acupuncturist's point of view, the Yin and Yang organs which are coupled to one another, such as liver and gall bladder or kidney and bladder, are so closely related that treatment of one will affect the other.

Case Histories. Two patients with chronic recurrent cystitis suffered from a constant dull ache over the bladder and often a burning pain on passing water. Treated with antibiotics the condition would be temporarily cured, only to reappear a few weeks or months later. One of the patients I treated by using bladder acupuncture points, the other by using only kidney acupuncture points. The result was equally good in both cases, as neither patient had more than minimal bladder trouble over the next few years.

In the above instance, treatment of either the Yin (kidney) or Yang (bladder) organ had the same result, showing the complete interdependence of the two. In other instances, however, stimulation of these two organs would not give the same result. This is where the skill of the doctor counts: he knows, given the circumstances, what will result from them.

PULSE DIAGNOSIS

The pulse diagnosis is the key-stone of Chinese traditional diagnosis. It is described in detail in the ancient treatises (Fig. 41).

'One should feel whether the pulse is in motion or whether it is still'.

'When the upper pulse is abundant, then the rebellious Qi rises. When the lower part is abundant, then the Qi causes a swelling in the abdomen. If the pulse appears to stop then the Qi has decayed.'

(Su Wen, Ch. 17)

'The "feon" pulse is like a weak wind that puffs up the feathers on the back of a bird, flustering and humming; like the wind that blows over autumn leaves; like water that moves the same swimming piece of wood up and down. . . .'

'If the pulse (at position III, left, deep) of the kidney is slightly hard . . . resistant . . . it is normal. If it is very hard, as hard as a stone, there will be death. . . .'

(Hübbotter, P. 179)

A doctor skilled in its practice would—without ever speaking to or seeing the face or body of his patient and with no more contact than a hand thrust through a hole in a curtain to give access to the radial artery of the wrist—be able to arrive at a reliable diagnosis in a matter of minutes.

It can be used to confirm a diagnosis already arrived at by clinical and laboratory methods. It can be of very great benefit in a case where, although the patient is obviously ill, it has not been possible to arrive at a conclusive diagnosis in spite of thorough clinical and laboratory investigations.

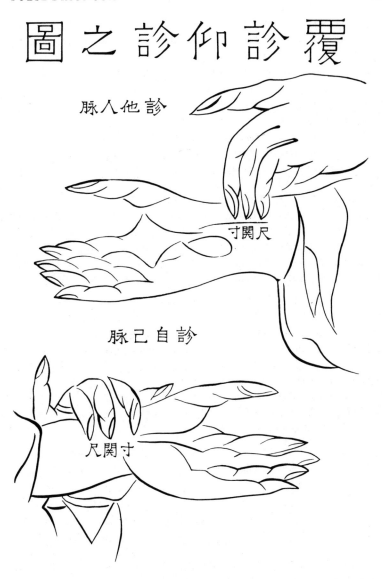

覆診仰診之圖

脉人他診

寸関尺

脉己自診

尺関寸

Fig. 41. Chinese pulse diagnosis, Sung dynasty. After Ilse Veith. The Yellow Emperor's Classic of Internal Medicine. 1949. Williams and Wilkins, Baltimore.

It is so sensitive a method of diagnosis that not too infrequently it will register past illnesses so accurately that a doctor is in a position to recount the past history of his patient's health (even though it involve illness he suffered fifty years previously) and to warn him of illness to be expected in the future, whether it be in several months' or in several years' time.

But such results as these can only be obtained under the correct conditions and within specific limitations, which must be strictly adhered to, so that not too much, nor too little, is expected of this method.

To those who do not understand its working, it can seem like magic. A patient who has been told by his doctor that at some time in the future he will develop a disease, though there is at the time no obvious indication to suggest it, may well conclude, when the 'prophecy' comes true, that his medical advisor has access to the secret mysteries of Nature.

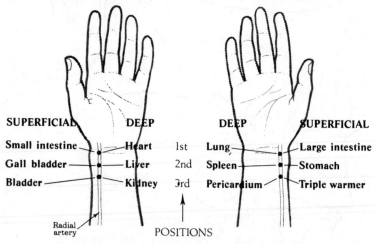

Fig. 42. The pulse diagnosis is the key to treatment.

To African Pygmies, utterly ignorant of the laws of aeronautics, an aeroplane taking flight like a giant bird above their heads, can only be explained in terms of magic. So we Europeans in our turn, observing some of the things the

Pygmies can do and being ignorant of the processes which make them possible, either dismiss them casually from our minds or apply to them that same word of 'magic'. In reality, both conclusions are no more than misconceptions and both are due to insufficient knowledge.

The pulse diagnosis is both a science and an art. The scheme in Fig. 42 describes how pulse diagnosis works, though in actual practice it can only be satisfactorily learnt by demonstration and continuous correction from a doctor who has mastered the technique.

The pulse at the radial artery of the wrist is divided into three zones, each of which has a superficial and a deep position.

Left hand			**Right hand**	
Superficial	*Deep*		*Deep*	*Superficial*
		Positions		
Small intestine	Heart	1st	Lung	Large intestine
Gall bladder	Liver	2nd	Spleen	Stomach
Bladder	Kidney	3rd	Pericardium	Triple warmer

Each position occupies about half an inch of the radial artery—the exact amount can only be judged when one has become practised in this art, as it varies in each individual. The second position is roughly opposite to the radial apophysis.

If the ball of the finger is lightly placed on the radial artery in these three positions, it will be noticed, except in a perfectly healthy person, that the sensation is different at each place, and if gradually a greater pressure is exerted, suddenly a point is reached where the sensation has a totally different quality. This is the deep position. The superficial position has been compared to the elasticity of the arterial wall, and the deep position to the sensation of the flow of blood within the artery. It has been suggested that the pressure required for the superficial pulse diagnosis is the diastolic pressure, while that for the deep pulse diagnosis is the systolic pressure.

A patient who has, for example, a duodenal ulcer, as demonstrated both clinically and by X-ray, will show a disturbance on the pulse marked 'stomach', i.e. the second position, superficial, right. Similarly, as discussed later, other diseases show on other pulses, though not always with an obvious correlation.

Case History. A girl with asthma missed so many of her lessons that discussions were in progress about sending her to a special school for the handicapped. From the point of view of acupuncture asthma may be due to a dysfunction of the lung or spleen or heart or kidney or liver, or it may be a non-specific type. Each one of the above six varieties has to be treated differently, and the pulse diagnosis is one of the best methods of differentiation. In this case the spleen was at fault, which when treated cured her asthma.

The Various Qualities

1. The pulse is different in every individual. There is no absolute norm, and something that may be normal for one individual, is pathological for another. Thus, the basic fundamental norm for each individual must be judged from experience, otherwise an attempt could be made to correct something which is normal so that disease would result.

It is, for example, perfectly normal for certain people to be vivacious and quick, and this is reflected in the quality of the radial pulse. For others, it is more normal to be of a phlegmatic temperament, and this is again reflected at the radial pulse. If an attempt be made to apply an artificial standard norm, to 'correct' these different (but in each case normal) pulses by 'appropriate' sedating or tonifying acupuncture points, disease will result. It is, after all, normal for an African to be black and a European to be white—an albino African is ill.

2. All the pulses in ensemble may be plethoric, in which all the twelve basic pulses beat too strongly and feel over-full. This is known as 'total plethora of Yin and Yang'.

All the superficial pulses in ensemble may be plethoric. This is called 'total plethora of Yang'.

All the deep pulses in ensemble may be plethoric. This is 'total plethora of Yin'.

3. All the pulses in ensemble may be much too weak. This may be called 'total weakness of Yin and Yang'.

Similarly we have:

'total weakness of Yang', and

'total weakness of Yin'.

4. If the pulses in position I are more powerful than the pulses in position III, Yang is more powerful than Yin. Similarly, if position III is stronger that position I, Yin is in excess of Yang.

5. If the pulses on the right artery are stronger than those on the left radial artery, there is excess of Yang. Conversely, if those on the left are stronger than those on the right, there is an excess of Yin.

Specific Qualities

Classically there are twenty-eight different qualities, though less than this is sufficient for ordinary practice.

'When the pulse of the spleen is soft and even, well separated, as the footsteps of a chicken touching the ground; it is called regular. When the pulse is full, the frequency increases, like a chicken lifting its feet; then one speaks of disease'.

(Jia Yi Jing, Vol. IV, Ch. 1a)

What might be called an artistic sense is a prerequisite for some of the finer points in pulse diagnosis, as frequently pulse conditions are felt which have not been felt before, or are not described in books.

Essentially the pulse acquires the same quality (in an artistic sense) as the organ which it represents. For example, I once felt the pulse of a doctor who did not tell me his symptoms or the result of investigations. The pulse of his stomach was like thickened, wet, soggy, blotting paper. I was unable to think of the diagnosis (it obviously being not a stomach ulcer, carcinoma or hyperacidity). The doctor then told me that he had, as diagnosed gastroscopically, hyper-trophic gastritis. The similarity (artistically speaking) between a hypertrophic gastric mucosa (the thickened lining of the stomach) and thickened, wet soggy, blotting paper are obvious. If my imagination had been a little livelier at the time, I am sure that I could have made the full diagnosis without the doctor concerned saying anything (Fig. 43).

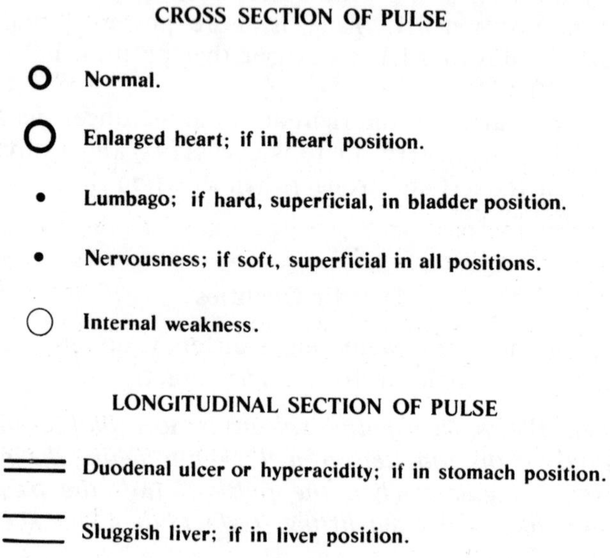

CROSS SECTION OF PULSE

O   Normal.

O   Enlarged heart; if in heart position.

•   Lumbago; if hard, superficial, in bladder position.

•   Nervousness; if soft, superficial in all positions.

○   Internal weakness.

LONGITUDINAL SECTION OF PULSE

▬▬   Duodenal ulcer or hyperacidity; if in stomach position.

▬▬   Sluggish liver; if in liver position.

Fig. 43. A few examples of pulse diagnosis.

1. A particular quality developed on only one flank of the same radial artery in the same position. e.g. a plethoric heart pulse which is more marked on the left side (lateral), suggests (to those who also think they can differentiate) that the left side of the heart is more strained than the right as is usual in hypertension.

2. The disturbance in the proximal or distal part of the pulse is more marked. For example in the case of the pulse of the large intestine, a disturbance in the distal part of the pulse is suggestive of disease of the anus, rectum or descend-ing colon; of the middle part, of the transverse colon; and the

proximal part of the pulse for the ascending colon. These qualities are difficult to appreciate.

3. A healthy person is one in whom the pulse flows smoothly, without turbulences or kinks, which has a certain tension but is yet compressible and elastic, and which has the same characteristics throughout its depth (Fig. 44 left).

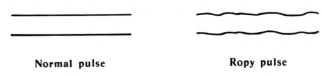

Normal pulse   Ropy pulse

Fig. 44.

A person who has a pulse like that described above is, physiologically speaking, perfectly healthy: if he has had diseases in the past, they have become fully healed, nor has he any latent diseases which are due to become active and develop obvious symptoms, giving objective findings. This type of person is not likely to have any serious illness and will probably live a long time. If he becomes ill there will be a disturbance in only one or two places on the pulse; this disturbed pulse position, whatever other qualities it may have, retains its elasticity, signifying that the disease can relatively easily be cured. If a diseased pulse position has a certain hard and brittle quality, the disease is harder to cure.

It is taught that on occasions in the course of a serious disease and shortly before death, the pulses become normal.

Only on rare occasions have I myself felt a perfectly normal pulse in someone who was ill. This illustrates that although the pulse is accurate to an astonishingly high degree it is not, any more than anything else, a hundred per cent foolproof. For this reason, and as a double check, it is usually advisable to take a history, make a physical examination, laboratory investigations, etc. as suggested by the individual case.

A history, physical examination and laboratory investigations are useful in directing one's attention to what one might expect to find on pulse diagnosis. So much may be found on the pulse that it is useful to have some other means to act as a pointer in discriminating between their relative importance. It should not be forgotten that the pulse divides diseases into twelve basic categories—and no more.

4. Diseases whether they be physical, physiological or mental show themselves on the pulse, provided the disease has a physiological effect.

If, for example, someone has had tuberculosis of the lungs, which has been fully healed so that the physiological function of the lungs is perfectly normal, the pulse of the lungs will be normal, despite the fact that a chest X-ray may show a few healed scars in the substance of the lungs. The pulse is normal because the scars (unless extensive) do not influence the physiological function (and hence health and disease) of the lungs; just as the physiological function of the skin is not influenced (to any appreciable degree) by the healed scars of a few minor skin abrasions. If the tuberculosis were still active, or the healed scars so extensive as to influence pulmonary function, it would show on the pulse.

A diabetic will, if untreated, have an abnormal pulse. If his pulse is felt at such an interval after taking insulin that his blood sugar-insulin balance is perfect, the pulse will be so near to normal, that an abnormality will be missed unless one is specifically looking for it. If the pulse is felt a few hours before or after this ideal insulin balance, the abnormality of the pulse will be detected more easily, though of course not as easily as in the uncontrolled diabetic.

A substantial proportion of mental diseases, contrary to certain opinion, is really physiological, and hence can be treated by acupuncture. It is, for example, well known that anyone who is livery is liable to be depressed, in which case the depression can be cured by treating the liver. (The liver symptoms may not be present, but show themselves on the pulse of the liver.) A depression which has a purely circumstantial cause (e.g. bankruptcy) does not show itself on the pulse. Mental diseases are discussed in detail elsewhere.

5. A pulse which is ropy in outline (Fig. 44 right) and consistency is a sign of general, chronic, physiological unbalance. People with this type of pulse are very difficult to cure.

If a person who has enjoyed good health for most of his life becomes ill, the pulse of the diseased organ becomes abnormal, while the pulses as a whole, remain normal and smooth.

The person with a ropy pulse may not even have a specific disease that can be localised, though as a rule it occurs in people who, for many years, have taken drugs in excessive amounts, or whose habit of living has included anything else that might undermine their general health. Sometimes a ropy pulse occurs in elderly people who have had many illnesses affecting several bodily systems, all of which have been only partly cured.

6. The hollow pulse. Certain pulses are hollow, the examining finger feeling a normal resistance on light application, but immediately greater pressure is applied the finger, as it were, falls through into a hollow. This pulse signifies, in general, a deficiency state.

7. The wire pulse. Sometimes all the pulses, or only the superficial or deep, or even an isolated pulse become taut, hard and thin, like the E string of a violin.

This pulse signifies spasm and pain. In a patient who has pain or spasm, it is natural to tighten up, which also occurs in the pulse which becomes hard and tight like a wire.

The wire pulse is typically seen on the bladder pulse in lumbago or sciatica. Nervous people may have all their superficial pulses wiry.

8. A hard, round, incompressible pulse, usually signifies a stone, whether it be biliary or renal. Occasionally the size of the stone can be judged in this way, and if it is judged small enough to be able to pass along the biliary ducts, the gall bladder may be stimulated to expel it.

9. A blown up pulse may occur in the stomach due to aerogastria; similarly the cardiac pulse may be blown up in cardiac strain or hypertrophy.

10. A coarse and rough pulse may be the result of cold weather. This condition disappears after the patient has been in a warm room for about half an hour.

11. The pulses become deeper in winter and in diseases associated with hardening and cold.

12. The pulses are more superficial in the summer and in febrile diseases.

13. Sometimes the pulse may be split longitudinally in two, which is more often noticed with the pulse of the gall bladder than with any other. I do not know the significance of this characteristic apart from the fact that it is associated with weakness. Possibly it indicates a non-synchronisation of the functions of the left and right biliary systems.

The Method of Utilising Physiological and Other Relationships

The more one feels the twelve basic pulses, the more does one have the impression that what is felt is not the specific organ concerned, such as the heart or the liver, but rather the basic 'conception' behind it, rather like Goethe's idea of the 'Urpflanze'.

Though obviously more than twelve organs or parts of the body can be effected by disease, with extremely few exceptions, they all show on the twelve basic pulses.

I think this can best be understood if the human being is considered as being in essence the result of the interplay of twelve basic forces which, in the course of embryonic development (and phylogenetic evolution), arrange the different individual cells and groups of cells to form twelve basic physiological and anatomical entities. The way that cells or groups of cells move during embryonic development along the most complicated paths is suggestive of some underlying force directing their movements. Embryologists explain this by the concepts of chemotaxis or polarity but these are probably only a very partial answer. Perhaps this can best be made clear by an example similar to that mentioned previously:

A disturbance in the liver pulse may be caused by:

(*a*) Disease of the liver itself—congestion, cirrhosis, carcinoma, etc.

(b) Haemorrhoids—the portal circulation, of which the haemorrhoidal veins are a part, passes through the liver. Hepatic congestion should always be treated first and only later the safety valve—the haemorrhoids.

(c) People who bruise easily. Presumably the clotting factors, such as prothrombim, are not sufficiently produced by a weak liver.

(d) Biliousness, nausea and vomiting.

(e) Migraine. Migraine (the usual type) is generally basically due to liver (and gall bladder) disturbance with the associated nausea. Most people with migrainous types of headache are first bilious and then some years later develop migraine.

(f) Weak eyesight, pain in or behind or around the eyes, black spots in front of eyes, zig-zags, etc. This may be explained via the traditional relationship between the eye and the liver (see chapter on five elements).

(g) Excessive muscular tension, especially around the shoulders and neck (see chapter of five elements) (Fig. 45).

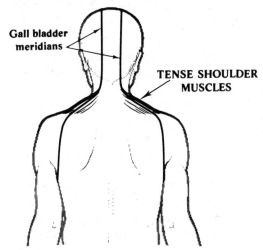

Fig. 45. Due to mental tension the shoulder muscles may tighten. The gall bladder meridian runs over these muscles; and hence the gall bladder or its coupled organ the liver, should be treated to relax the muscles.

(*h*) Inability to wake up fresh in the morning, however early one has gone to bed (Fig. 14).

(*i*) Certain types of asthma, hay fever, skin rashes and other allergic or 'stress' symptoms. Probably due to manufacture of antibodies and other factors in the liver (Fig. 46).

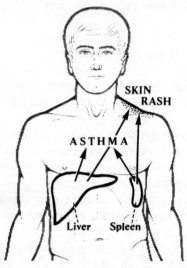

Fig. 46. The liver (and spleen) manufacture antibodies, and their respective meridians can be treated in certain allergic asthmas or skin rashes.

The above-mentioned diseases may cause the disturbance of other pulses in addition to that of the liver. In addition most diseases have various causes, some of which will not affect the liver and therefore will not register on the liver pulse.

There are, of course, many more diseases which register as a disturbance on the pulse of the liver, but for the purposes of this discussion no more need be mentioned.

It will be noticed that most of the diseases or symptoms mentioned above (*a*) to (*i*) are related (whether it be physiologically, anatomically, or by various laws of acupuncture) to the liver. The liver is the one factor that unites all these diseases, even though some of them may superficially not seem to have any relation to one another.

Similarly, if all the diseases of mankind are considered (excluding those few that have no physiological effect), it will be found that they all cause the alteration of one or several of the twelve basic pulses, and are hence related to the twelve basic organs. Anyone who is able to carry out the pulse diagnosis accurately, may prove the above statement to himself.

This fundamental conception that the human being is divisible into twelve basic physiological systems, to which other factors are subservient, is a gift for which we are indebted to the ancient Chinese of prehistoric times, for it is described in such detail in one of the oldest medical books in the world (The Nei Jing), that its origin must lie in a period that is even more remote.

When feeling the pulse, one has the impression, that what is felt is not the disease itself, but rather the entelechy behind the disease, showing itself only later as a disease in one or other branch of the basic twelve. This conception of the entelechy of disease is also suggested by the observation that the tendency to one of the basic twelve diseases can be foretold on the pulse diagnosis, months or even years before the disease or any symptoms or objective findings occur. This is the basic tendency which is only at a later date specialised into a specific disease.

FACTORS THAT SHOULD BE TAKEN INTO ACCOUNT WHEN PALPATING THE PULSE

Certain difficulties may be encountered in pulse diagnosis which may, in certain circumstances, necessitate relegating the pulse diagnosis to a secondary position (Fig. 47).

Naturally the easiest pulse to palpate is that of the healthy middle-aged person, where the pulse is fairly elastic. In little children care must be taken because of the smallness of the pulse. In the aged plaques of atheroma (a type of 'hardening of the arteries') in the radial artery may confuse the picture. It seems, as a rule, that if an atheromatous plaque is located specifically at a certain pulse position, then the organ system represented is diseased.

In certain people a dilation of the radial artery may occur at a particular pulse position. It might be considered that this dilation is merely secondary to a localised weakening of the radial artery and therefore dismissed. Experience usually

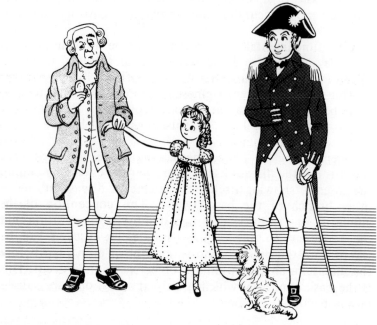

Fig. 47. In people with one arm, the pulse diagnosis cannot be done satisfactorily. Often though the symptoms of the patient are a sufficient guide. Pulse diagnosis done on a near blood relative may help, such as Nelson and his daughter Horatia.

shows, however, that the organ represented by the dilated segment is rather severly diseased and is fairly resistant to treatment.

In marked hypo- or hypertension the pulse is either so uniformly weak or strong, that individual characteristics are difficult to palpate, unless the hypo- or hypertension are first treated.

External influences must always be considered: Drugs, excessive food or drink, running, emotion, etc.

X

DISEASES THAT MAY BE TREATED BY ACUPUNCTURE

Theoretically it is possible to help or cure by acupuncture any disease that can be affected by a physiological process. Duodenal ulcer, acne vulgaris, migraine, for example, are all the result of physiological process, and as such may be cured: the duodenal ulcer, by reducing the amount of acid produced by the stomach; the acne, by increasing the function of the lungs and hormonal regulation; the migraine, by increasing the function of the liver.

A trouble that is purely anatomical and uninfluencable by a physiological process, such as a kidney stone, advanced osteoarthritis, a fully formed cataract, cannot be treated by this means. Human physiology is such that it is hardly ever possible for destructive changes in bones to be repaired—though it is obviously possible to affect the circulation and swelling around an arthritic joint, without though altering the bone very much. In a cataract the protein of the lens of the eye has become denatured (as the transparent part of an egg becomes white when it is boiled), a chemical change that cannot be reversed under the normal conditions of life.

The capacity for the regeneration of the new tissue in the human being must be taken into account when judging the possibility of a cure. It must be remembered that the human has less power of regeneration than any animal, and vastly less than the lower animals. A flat worm will completely regenerate itself if it is cut in half longitudinally or transversely (so that two flat worms are made out of one); if the tail of a rain worm is cut off, it will partially regrow; the fin of a lung fish will grow again if it has been broken off; similarly the limbs of an amphibia (if cut under experimental conditions). The human organism has not this same regenerative power. His creative energy has been transferred to the power of thought.

From the point of view of Chinese medicine, there is often no essential difference between a physical and a mental disease, for in theory:

1 A physical dysfunction can cause a mental disease.
2 A mental dysfunction can cause a physical disease.
3 A physical dysfunction can cause a physical disease.
4 A mental dysfunction can cause a mental disease.

To give an example:

(a) If someone lives in depressing circumstances for a short time, then the depressing circumstances effect his mode of thinking, and he becomes depressed. If after a *short* while the depressing circumstances disappear, then the patient can usually readjust himself mentally and the depression disappears.

(b) If on the other hand the depressing circumstances continue for a *long* time, then the depressed mind of the patient will eventually affect the liver (see relation between the liver and depression in the chapter on the five elements). Once the liver is affected, even if the original depressing circumstances are removed, the depression will remain. This depression can only be cured if the liver is treated—provided the depressing external circumstances have also been removed (Fig. 48).

(c) If someone harms his liver, by for example eating a poison that destroys part of the liver, then the patient may (i) have predominantly physical symptoms such as jaundice, an abdomen full of ascitic fluid or an itching skin, or he may (ii) have predominantly mental symptoms such as depression or an uncontrollable anger. In this instance whether the patient has physical or mental symptoms the liver would have to be treated physically.

To take another example of a mental disease which is really a physical disease and can therefore be treated by acupuncture: Most people who have various disturbances which include fear have an underactivity of the kidney (many frightened children are bed wetters—kidney; after a fright most people wish to pass urine—kidney). Actors with stage fright, teachers with lack of confidence, others before interviews, examinations, driving tests, people who are afraid to leave their house to meet strangers—all these are often kidney weaknesses which may be cured by treating the kidney. The law of the five elements, described earlier, indicates which organ is the culprit for the main categories of mental diseases.

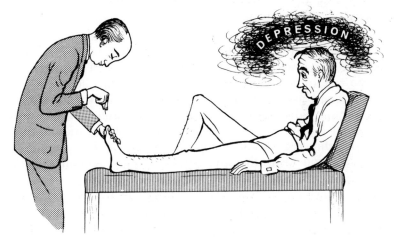

Fig. 48. A prick in the big toe may cure a depression.

Case History. A regular colonel whom I saw in my consulting rooms had left the army at 45 and had to start civilian life. This involved interviews with many prospective employers. A certain degree of nervousness would be normal under the circumstances, but he was excessively nervous, so that he became unbearable at home. Pulse diagnosis showed an underactive kidney, which when treated reduced the excessive nervous tension, to one of normal proportions.

Case History. During the course of a takeover bid a patient's nerves were so shattered that he started shaking to such an extent that he could not pour out a cup of tea. The whole takeover bid was from his point of view jeopardised by his excessive nervous reaction, shaking hands, sleeplessness, fits of suicidal depression etc. In his instance there was a dysfunction of the lung and heart which was quickly cured, and I am glad to say the patient's part of the firm prospered. He thanked me afterwards especially as he had been dragged to see me against his will by his wife.

One of the great contributions of Chinese medicine is the ability to link physical and mental diseases, whereby it is often found that a physical disease has a mental cause, and a mental disease a physical cause. In either case they may be treated by acupuncture.

In acupuncture psychologists would have a powerful weapon with which to treat their patients in a rational manner instead of rolling tranquilisers down their throats, passing electric currents through their brains, or discussing those parts of their sex life which they would rather forget. The role of the psychologist will still remain though in what has been classified above as (2) a mental dysfunction causing a physical disease and (4) a mental dysfunction causing a mental disease. Quite apart from the above considerations a good clinician should know which method (tranquilisers, electric convulsive therapy, psycho-analysis, acupuncture etc) to apply in a given case.

The list of illnesses given below may be found in most books on acupuncture; some authors mention more, some less. Among the diseases listed some may be cured in nearly every case treated, while others may only yield to treatment in a small proportion of the patients treated. The duration of the disease, the amount of damage done, the general constitution of the individual patient must be taken into account. In many diseases, which have progressed too far for it to be possible to effect a cure, it is often possible to arrest the disease so that it does not progress any further; or a disease which is severely incapacitating may, at least, be partially cured or relieved, so that the man or woman may continue living a reasonably normal life.

Vague feelings of malaise, not feeling 100% fit but not really ill, not having enough energy or drive, etc., etc., are really all pre-clinical symptoms of disease, which, if they persist long enough, will quite likely result in actual disease.

These vague preclinical symptoms can usually be precisely recognised by the pulse diagnosis (as discussed in the chapter on Preventive Medicine), and immediately treated. The increased sense of both physical and mental well-being that may thus be achieved, is a major contribution of acupuncture.

It is often said that 'the patient's psyche does not matter'. This is not true. It is not true for ordinary medicine nor for acupuncture, though some people (I think quite erroneously) consider that an objective diagnosis cannot be made unless the thoughts and feelings of both patient and doctor are disregarded, and a medical consultation is conducted like a test-tube experiment. It is well known to anaesthetists that the dose of anaesthetic required, especially for light anaesthesia, may have to be either doubled or halved according to the mental attitude of the patient—whether he wishes to become unconscious or whether he resists. The speed of recovery after an operation or the chances of life or death for a person who is very seriously ill are, as most doctors will agree from their own experience, partly a matter of the will power of the patient.

It is sometimes assumed that the mind is subjective, irresponsible and unreal, a negligible factor in medicine, since it cannot be measured; while the body is objective, measurable and real. To the acupuncturist they are but two facets of the same problem. Under certain circumstances one facet is more important, while at other times the other.

Some who have not experienced or seen the results of acupuncture get the impression that it is little more than hypnotism. This is by no means the case for:

(a) Acupuncture will work if the patient is completely unconscious under a general anaesthetic.

(b) There are certain sensitive people who notice the effect of a needle within a few seconds. As an acupuncture point is small it is occasionally possible to miss the exact spot, whereupon the sensitive patient, if he has already had experience of the treatment, will remark that it is not working. The acupuncturist can verify this by the pulse diagnosis. This should, in any case, be repeated as a routine after all the acupuncture needles are in place, for the pulse should alter within seconds of the needle being put in. If the needle is then readjusted by one tenth of an inch the sensitive patient will at once feel the difference, which may be verified by the pulse diagnosis.

(c) Occasional cases of spontaneous cures may be attributed to accidental injuries to acupuncture points. This is rarely the case as at any one time only a few acupuncture points are active—and they are small. An injury over a large area which may include one or several acupuncture points seems to have no specific effect. The stimulus must be localised to have an effect.

Tropical disease, of which most European acupuncturists have no practical experience are not mentioned in the index.

Various acute surgical emergencies such as appendicitis, peritonitis, etc. and various other potentially lethal diseases are not mentioned in the index, for although the acupuncturist may well be able to treat them (as is done in China today), most European acupuncturists will, as a matter of principle, not treat these diseases, as acupuncture is new to Europe. In addition, many of these acute emergencies can be well treated by orthodox medicine.

'Some people say one cannot cure a chronic disease. This though is quite wrong. An expert acupuncturist may cure it as easily as: taking out a thorn, or wiping away snow flakes, or untying a knot, or pulling out a cork. Even if a disease is of long duration it can be cured; those who say it is incurable do not know acupuncture properly.'

(Jia Yi Jing, Vol. II, Ch. 1a)

Duration of Treatment

The number of treatments required to effect a cure varies considerably. The average patient when seen by the acupuncturist for the first time does not, as a rule, have merely one disease, but in addition a variety of mild chronic complaints which do not incapacitate him, but simply make life less pleasant. It is a flare-up of these mildly chronic ailments that actually brings the sufferer to the doctor. The patient may have, for example, dyspepsia, a bitter taste in the mouth, frequent headaches, insomnia, brittle nails, and an irritable mood that he cannot control. One or more of these symptoms will have become acute; for instance, the dyspepsia may have developed into a duodenal ulcer.

All these symptoms (in one individual patient) including the duodenal ulcer, will take an average of about seven treatments to cure (or if a cure is not possible, to ameliorate).

Once a patient has been completely cured of his various ailments and the pulse is normal, provided he is seen by the doctor for a check-up every six months (as described in the chapter on preventive medicine), his basic health will then, as a rule, remain satisfactory. If he should then (with a basically sound health) develop an illness it can usually be cured in relatively few treatments—even a single one sometimes being sufficient.

Certain difficult diseases, especially if they have been in existence over a substantial portion of the patient's life, have a hereditary tendency or have resulted in anatomical changes, may easily take more than seven treatments to cure.

A disease of short duration, provided the causes, which may not be apparent, are also of short duration, will probably take less than seven treatments.

A very small proportion of patients who do not improve while they are being treated, may notice an amelioration or even a cure some months later—seemingly the healing process can be very slow.

Response to Treatment

The speed of response varies considerably from patient to patient, and with each disease.

Certain patients feel a response within a few seconds of the first needles being in place the first time they come for treatment. Others may have to be treated four or possibly even more times, for the first response to be felt (Fig. 49).

The effect of a single treatment may be noticed during the treatment or several hours or days later.

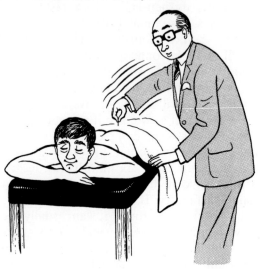

Fig. 49. Treatment in progress.

After a treatment nothing tangible may be noticed. At other times there may be an increase in energy, a lightness and buoyancy due to the stimulating effect of the treatment (Fig. 50). In some people there is a great feeling of relaxation which may be followed by a pleasant drowsiness due to the sudden release of tension.

Occasionally, and in certain people, there is a reaction before the improvement starts. This may seem, if it is not understood, to be a worsening of the condition. A reaction may be compared to what happens in the case of an infection deep in the hand which first becomes an acute boil (seemingly a worsening of the condition—the reaction) before it discharges its accumulated pus to the exterior. The infection in the hand could also have been cured by the absorption of the infection into the blood stream. In the latter case the improvement would have progressed smoothly without a reaction. With or without a reaction the end result is the same, though the acupuncturist naturally always tries to effect a cure the smooth way. Certain chronic conditions

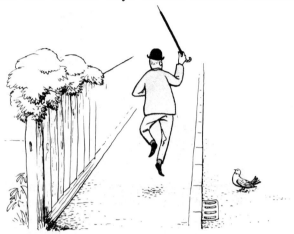

Fig. 50. A lightness and buoyancy after acupuncture treatment.

however have, of necessity, to be brought to an acute stage (the reaction) for it to be possible to cure them. On rare occasions a reaction may be experienced after every treatment. The following letter illustrates a rather extreme example.

Dear Dr. Mann,   26.3.70
    The effects of your last treatment were so extraordinary I think you'd like to know about them!
    For 48 hours I suffered a great deal of severe pain—codis* twice in the night and once or twice next day failed to ease it and my spine and neck and back got worse and worse.
    At one moment on the second day I thought I was going to seize up as I've done before and I thought 'I *must* get to Dr. Mann' for a needling, only to be brought short by remembering it was the needling that had brought it on.

* A pain killer.

Then it passed and steadily I improved till every one of the symptoms—waves of nausea, livery-ishness, pains† went and even, for the first time in years, I found myself able to drink an ordinary amount of wine (strongly disapproved of for me by my medico's who prefer that I take 'purple hearts') without any subsequent heaviness or other liver symptoms.

'Cheers!' Well done and thank you very much!

With all good wishes from a grateful and rejuvenated old lady.

Yours sincerely.

The improvement that is noticed during a course of acupuncture does not follow a steady course. As a rule the degree of improvement and its duration increases with each treatment till the stage is reached where the improvement persists and becomes a cure that lasts. The improvement from the first treatment may last minutes, hours or days, the effect lasting longer with each repetition. Some patients improve rapidly at the beginning of treatment but may take a long time to achieve that extra little bit that makes the cure; others improve slowly at the beginning and then take a sudden turn and are cured in no time. The majority follow an intermediate course. Most often there are various ups and downs during treatment and there is rarely an absolutely steady improvement—nature does not know straight lines. Not infrequently there is a setback at some stage of the treatment, which is then overcome by altering the acupuncture points used.

The final result rests with the individual doctor, his knowledge and ability.

A list (admittedly incomplete) of diseases that may be cured or helped is given below. In any individual case a certain disease may better be treated by orthodox medicine or in combination with orthodox medicine or by other means. The best course can only be decided in dealing with an actual case.

† She was unable to walk far.

HEAD
Neuralgia, headaches, migraine, fainting, trigeminal neuralgia (sometimes), tics, spasms.

LIMBS AND MUSCULATURE
Fibrositis, muscular rheumatism, sciatica, lumbago, swelling, discoloration, cramps, intermittent claudication, cold hands and feet (sometimes), oedema, writers' cramp, weakness, some types of trembling, neuralgia of shoulders and arms, tennis elbow, early rheumatoid or osteoarthritis, weakness or feeling of excessive heaviness of limbs, frozen shoulder.

DIGESTION
Duodenal ulcer, hyperacidity, gastritis, dyspepsia, inability to eat ordinary food, non-digestion of food, no appetite, undigested stools, pale stools, eructation, wind, abdominal distension, bad breath, dry mouth, bad taste in mouth, heartburn, pyloric spasm, nausea, vomiting, diarrhoea, various types of colic, underfunction of liver, tender liver, chronic cholecystitis, colitis, pancreatitis, nausea and vomiting of pregnancy, vomiting of children and infants, abdomen feels cold.

RESPIRATORY SYSTEM
Asthma, bronchitis, tracheitis, shortness of breath, pulmonary congestion, recurrent colds, coughs and mild pulmonary infections.

CARDIO VASCULAR SYSTEM
Angina pectoris, pseudo angina pectoris, pain or heaviness over cardiac area, fainting, palpitations, tachycardia, arythmia, phlebitis, haemorrhoids, lymphangeitis, adenitis, pallor, pins and needles, poor circulation, fainting, feels easily cold.

GENITO URINARY SYSTEM
Cystitis, some types of renal colic, lumbago, bladder irritation and spasm, bed wetting, lack of control of bladder.

SEXUAL SYSTEM
Pelvic pain, painful periods, irregular periods, flooding, vaginal pain, itching, menopausal trouble, hot flushes, ovarian pain, mastitis, menopausal loss of hair (sometimes), tender breasts.

EYES
Weak eyesight, tired after reading a book a short time, not optical defects, black spots and zig-zags in front of eyes, pain behind or around eye, conjunctivitis, blepharitis.

EAR, NOSE AND THROAT
Hay fever, rhinitis, nose bleeding, sneezing, loss of smell (some types), sinusitis, tonsillitis, laryngitis, loss of voice, pharyngitis, Menières syndrome.

SKIN
Acne, itching, eczema, urticaria, abscesses, herpes, neurodermatitis, etc.

NERVOUS SYSTEM AND PSYCHIATRIC FACTORS
Nervousness, depression, anxiety, fears, obsessions, timidity, stage fright, neurasthenia, wish to die, agitation, outbursts of temper, yawning, excessive loquacity, sleeplessness, nocturnal, terror, many neuralgias, neuralgia after shingles (sometimes), petit mal (sometimes), trembling, trigeminal neuralgia (sometimes).

GENERAL STATE
General fatigue, lassitude, excessive perspiration, excessive sleep, excessive yawning, sensitive to changes in temperature, travel sickness, post operative weakness after severe diseases, insomnia, post-viral fatigue or myalgic encephalomyelitis.

CHILDREN

Many of the more common diseases of children, excepting the infectious disease. Children respond quickly. An important aim of acupuncture is to achieve and maintain healthy childhood, as much illhealth of later years can then be avoided. Bed-wetting, fear of the dark, bad tempered or frightened states, inability to learn properly at school, under-development, stunted growth (sometimes), cyclic vomiting and acidosis infants, lack of appetite.

GENERAL HEALTH

Most patients who have been treated by acupuncture notice a considerable improvement in their general health. This is because acupuncture can correct those minor disturbances in health which are undetected by other methods of diagnosis, and which if they remained untreated could in later years turn into an overt and easily recognised disease. The sensitivity of Chinese pulse diagnosis (see chapter on Preventive Medicine) makes it possible to detect minor disturbances, enabling immediate treatment to be given at an early stage.

The above list of diseases might seem to some people rather long, as if acupuncture were to be regarded as a general panacea. It should be realised however that acupuncture is not a single drug, such as penicillin, which is therapeutically applicable to only a limited variety of infections. It is, on the contrary, a whole system of medicine which encompasses many dysfunctions of the body. Hence the title of this book.

Some of the illnesses or symptoms mentioned above may be helped in a high proportion of patients, whilst others only in a moderate, small or very small proportion. Orthodox medicine is, of course, not infrequently the best answer. The success of much of acupuncture depends on many individual factors which an expert should usually be able to assess at the first consultation.

XI

PREVENTIVE MEDICINE

In ancient China a first class physician was one who could not only cure disease but could also prevent disease. Only a second class physician had to wait until his patients became ill so that he could then treat them when there were obvious symptoms and signs.

It is for this reason that the doctor was paid by the patient when he was healthy and the payment was stopped when he was ill. This was so much so that the doctor had to give the patient free of cost the medicines required, medicines which he, the doctor, had paid for out of his own pocket.

'To administer medicines to diseases which have already developed and to supress revolts which have already developed is comparable to the behaviour of those persons who begin to dig a well after they have become thirsty, and of those who begin to make their weapons after they have already engaged in battle. Would these actions not be too late?'

(Su Wen, Ch. 2)

This type of preventive medicine (Fig. 51) is based in acupuncture on the pulse diagnosis, which, as already mentioned, presents in its early stages, rather the entelechy of disease than the disease itself.

It is well known that the person who will at a later date develop, for instance, hypertension, exhibits certain mental symptoms (a certain stiff walk and fixedness of ideas), many years before the hypertension as such shows itself and similarly with other diseases. This type of preclinical symptomatology is so vague and uncertain that, on the whole, little use can be made of it.

The pulse diagnosis, on the other hand, is a relatively certain indication of preclinical disease. A little consideration will show that before a disease develops with physical signs and objective findings, there will be, possibly for months or years beforehand, some physiological disturbance that is too slight to cause overt symptoms. But, even at this stage, the pulse registers a definite abnormality.

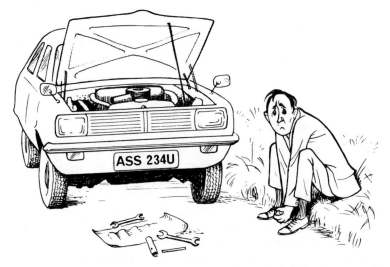

Fig. 51. Do you service your car (or body) regularly? Or do you wait till you have trouble?

The acupuncturist will at this preclinical stage treat the patient, using acupuncture points dictated to him solely by the pulse diagnosis.

For preventive medicine of this type to be effective, the patient must, of course, see the doctor at regular intervals. In my experience a person with a reasonable constitution need only have his pulse felt every six months; which is the same interval at which one should visit a dentist. Once a year is enough for the exceptionally healthy.

One additional advantage of this preventive routine is that the whole general level of health is maintained at a higher level. It can give not only the absence of disease, but a positive feeling of well-being with an abundance of physical and mental energy.

Very often people are not actually ill, but feel a little below what they sense should be ideal health. This is, in reality, the preclinical stage of disease which may take very many years till it is seen as an overt disease. If this person is correctly treated, not only is the slight fatigue, etc. cured, but in addition he is spared the consequences of later developing an obvious disease.

The Yellow Emperor once addressed T'ien Shih, the divinely inspired teacher: *'I have heard that in ancient times the people lived to be over a hundred years, and yet they remained active and did not become decrepit in their activities. But nowadays people only reach half of that age and yet become decrepit and failing. Is it that mankind is degenerating through the ages and loses its original vigour?'*

Qi Bo, the chief physician, answered: *'In ancient times those people who understood the ways of nature, patterned themselves upon the Yin and the Yang. . . .'*

(Su Wen, Ch. 1)

For preventive acupuncture to be effective, the initial treatment must have been successful, so that the pulse has become normal. It may not be possible to completely cure someone who has been ill for many years; though the patient may say he is cured as he has no symptoms. In this case the pulse will still show a slight abnormality which cannot be corrected. In this type preventive acupuncture is only partially effective. If the patient had been seen earlier, preventive acupuncture would have been fully effective.

We have to face the fact that, in our modern civilization, with its many influences which are detrimental to health, by no means all diseases can be prevented. Preventive medicine applies particularly to the chronic and degenerative diseases and not to such an extent to the infective diseases or those caused by external agents, except insofar as the general resistance has been increased.

Various additional factors should not be forgotten: Exercise, naturally grown food that is not poisoned or devitalised, good air, enough relaxation and enough thought (Fig. 52).

'Modern man drinks wine like water, leads an irregular life, engaging in sexual intercourse while he is drunk, thus exhausting his vital forces; they do not know how to preserve their vital forces, wasting their energy excessively, seeking

---

In a box from birth to death....

the similarity in the life of a battery chicken and man.

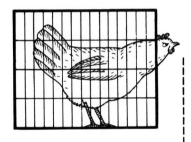 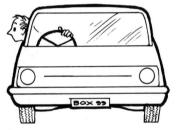

A battery chicken has little exercise, eats semi-artificial food and leads an unnatural life.

Their meat has an insipid taste, they are often sterile, and need many medicines to keep them alive.

Modern man tends to use the car and tin opener excessively.

What will be his fate?

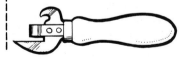

Fig. 52.

only physical pleasure, all of which is against the rules of nature. For these reasons they reach only one half of the hundred years and then they degenerate'.

(Su Wen, Ch. 1)

The above describes the traditional Chinese approach to preventive medicine. In my own practice I prefer a modification:

I normally see a patient initially for a specific illness or symptoms. Once I have cured these (if that is possible) and also cured any other condition the patient may have, the patient is discharged. If a patient has had the illness for a short while, the initial course of treatment is usually sufficient. If they have been ill for many years there may be a tendency for their symptoms to recur at longish intervals. One treatment is usually sufficient for these recurrences if they are mild, and therefore further development of the illness is prevented.

STATISTICS

On the whole, the following statistics, are in my opinion somewhat optimistic; though they may if diluted be used as a rough guide. I know of no statistics, in China or the West, which correspond with my present-day experience of acupuncture. I have little doubt, now that a greater number of doctors are practising acupuncture in the West, that more accurate statistics will in the ensuing years be published. These will be incorporated in later printings of this book.

It should not be forgotten that acupuncture is mainly suitable for diseases which are physiologically reversible, i.e. it may cure asthma; it may help (but not cure) the early stages of chronic bronchitis; whilst the later stages of chronic bronchitis, bronchietasis or emphysema are not helped except in so far as they have an element of spasm.

A

The following statistics of Mauries* (Marseille) may act as a guide. It consists of all (625) the patients he treated in a specified period who had been previously diagnosed and treated by doctors other than acupuncturists, with little or no success. It does not include patients who visited Dr Mauries before they had seen another doctor; so that the possible statistical error of a spontaneous cure despite treatment is at least partly negated. Patients whom he has not been able to contact, or who have left his district, have not been included. Despite the fact that the diagnosis has been made by at least two doctors in each case, it will be obvious

* (Actes des Ill eme Journees International d'Acupuncture).

to the reader that some of the criteria used in diagnosis and the meaning attached to a particular diagnosis are a little different from those usually employed in England, for which due allowance should be made.

Rheumatic and allied diseases	No. treated	Cured	Improved	Failure
Lumbago	29	19	6	4
Sciatica	25	15	4	6
Facial neuralgia	11	6	4	1
Rheumatism of several joints	36	19	11	6
P.C.E.	5	3	1	1
Cervical arthritis	9	5	3	1
Pain in heel of foot	2	2	—	—
Interscapular neuralgia	1	—	—	1
Gout of big toe	2	2	—	—
Tennis elbow	1	—	—	1
Osteo-arthritis	1	—	1	—
Generalised vertebral arthritis	3	2	1	—
Coccydynia	2	—	—	2
Arthritis of knee	14	9	1	4
Mandibular arthritis	2	1	—	1
Frozen shoulder	4	2	1	1
Rheumatism of knee and ankle	1	1	—	—
Coxarthritis	1	—	—	1
Intercostal neuralgia	3	2	—	1
Hernia of lumbar disc	1	—	—	1
Traumatic lumbar pain	1	—	—	1
Arthritis of shoulder	5	3	2	—
Cervico-brachial neuralgia	5	4	1	—
Post-menopausal rheumatism	1	1	—	—
Rheumatism of ankle	2	2	—	—
	167	98	36	33

i.e. 80% cured or improved.

Pulmonary diseases	No. treated	Cured	Improved	Failure
Hay fever	9	6	—	3
Emphysema	10	3	4	3
Chronic bronchitis	3	1	2	—
Asthma	38	24	8	6
Cough due to hypertension	1	1	—	—
	61	35	14	12

i.e. 80% cured or improved.

Urology	No. treated	Cured	Improved	Failure
Cystitis	2	2	—	—
Incontinence	8	2	3	3
Renal colic	1	1	—	—
	11	5	3	3

i.e. 72% cured or improved.

E.N.T.	No. treated	Cured	Improved	Failure
Streptomycin tinnitis	1	—	—	1
Chronic sinusitis	1	1	—	—
Chronic tracheitis	2	1	—	1
Chronic laryngitis	1	1	—	—
Chronic otorrhea	1	1	—	—
Catarrhal deafness	1	1	—	—
Allergic oedema of larynx	1	1	—	—
Post menopausal deafness	1	—	—	1
	9	6	0	3

i.e. 66% cured or improved.

Gynaecology	No. treated	Cured	Improved	Failure
Dysmenorrhea	5	5	—	—
Hypermenorrhea	1	1	—	—
Menstrual trouble	1	1	—	—
	7	7	0	0

i.e. 100% cured or improved.

Diseases of arteries and veins	No. treated	Cured	Improved	Failure
Arteritis of leg	3	–	2	1
Circulatory disturbance in a man	1	1	–	–
Circulatory disturbance in a woman	2	1	–	1
	6	2	2	2

i.e. 66% cured or improved.

Cardiology	No. treated	Cured	Improved	Failure
Cardiac asthma	2	–	–	2
Paroxysmal tachycardia	1	1	–	–
	3	1	0	2

i.e. 33% cured.

Digestive tract	No. treated	Cured	Improved	Failure
Gastralgia	3	3	–	–
Diarrhoea with food	1	1	–	–
Vomiting due to megaoesophagus	1	–	–	1
Peptic ulcer	1	1	–	–
Vomiting of infants	3	3	–	–
Chronic diarrhoea	2	2	–	–
Constipation	8	4	–	3
Biliary atony	6	5	1	–
Gastric ulcer	4	2	1	1
Habitual vomiting	1	1	–	–
Cholecystitis in a colonial	1	1	–	–
Gastralgia in a syphilitic	1	1	–	–
	32	25	2	5

i.e. 84% cured or improved.

Neurology	No. treated	Cured	Improved	Failure
Littles disease	1	–	1	–
Results of hemiplegia	6	–	5	1
Myelitis	1	–	–	1
Para-facial spasm of Meige	1	–	1	–
Epilepsy	1	–	1	–
Tabetic pains	1	1	–	–
Parkinson's disease	3	–	–	3
Atrophy due to polio	1	–	1	–
Spasmodic quadriplegia due to cervical disc	1	–	1	–
Disseminated sclerosis	3	–	–	3
	19	1	9	9

i.e. 52% of improvements including one cure.

Endocrinal diseases	No. treated	Cured	Improved	Failure
Diabetes mellitus	3	–	–	3
Diabetes insipidus	1	–	1	–
Hyperthyroidism	1	–	1	–
Too short in stature	1	–	1	–
Adrenal insufficiency	1	1	–	–
Pagets disease	1	–	1	–
	8	1	4	3

i.e. 62% cured or improved.

Neuro-vegetative disequilibrium (syncope, tachycardia, globus hystericus, spasms, lassitude, etc.)

	No. treated	Cured	Improved	Failure
General neuro-vegetative disequilibrium	208	151	23	34
Post operative functional disturbances	3	3	–	–
Nervous hypertension	12	11	1	–
Neurasthenia	5	2	2	1
Vomiting of pregnancy	1	1	–	–
Angina pectoris	2	2	–	–

Neuritis of pregnancy	1	–	–	1
Pruritis ani	1	–	–	1
Eczema	1	1	–	–
'Floaters'	1	–	–	1
Demencia praecox	1	1	–	–
Plexalgia	1	1	–	–
Yawning	2	2	–	–
Excessive sleepiness	1	1	–	–
	240	176	26	38

i.e. 84% cured or improved.

Diverse diseases	No. treated	Cured	Improved	Failure
Quincke's oedema	3	3	–	–
Taenia	1	1	–	–
Excessive loss of weight	2	2	–	–
Amyotrophia	1	–	1	–
Furunculosis	2	2	–	–
Hiccups	1	–	1	–
Idiopathic headaches	6	3	2	1
Aphthous stomatitis	1	–	–	1
Non cardiac oedema of ankles	1	–	–	1
Seborrhea	1	–	–	1
Asthenia and anaemia	2	2	–	–
Bad at mathematics	4	4	–	–
Vertigo	1	1	–	–
Psoriasis	1	–	–	1
Obesity in a woman	1	1	–	–
Ophthalmic herpes zosta	1	1	–	–
Insomnia	3	2	1	–
	32	22	5	5

i.e. 84% cured or improved.

B

The following statistics are taken from the Department of Surgery, Chung Shan Medical College, Canton, China*. They are concerned with the treatment of thirty-six cases of acute

* Chinese Medical Journal 79: 27-76, July, 1959.

appendicitis, ten of appendicular abscess and three of perforated appendix with general peritonitis. They were treated mainly by acupuncture; though ten of them were treated by traditional Chinese herbs or a combination of both methods.

1. DURATION AFTER ONSET OF ILLNESS

Duration	Acute appendicitis	Appendicular abscess	Perforated appendix
2-6 hours	5		
6-12 hours	5		
12-24 hours	9	1	
24-48 hours	5		2
48-72 hours	4	2	1
4 days	2	1	
6 days	1		
7 days		2	
8 days		1	
10 days		1	
15 days		2	
Records unavailable	5		
	36	10	3

2. TEMPERATURE ON ADMISSION

Temperature	Acute appendicitis		Appendicular abscess		Perforated appendix
Normal	11				
High	24		9		3
37.1-38°C		17		3	
38.1-39°C		5		6	3
39.1-40°C		2			
Records unavailable	1		1		
	36		10		3

3. W.B.C. ON ADMISSION

W.B.C.	Acute appendicitis	Appendicular abscess	Perforated appendix
7,000 or less	4	–	–
7,000-10,000	8	1	–
10,000-20,000	19	6	2
20,000-30,000	1	2	1
30,000-40,000	1	–	–
Records unavailable	3	1	–
	36	10	3

4. SYMPTOMS AND SIGNS OF ACUTE APPENDICITIS CASES BEFORE TREATMENT

	No. of cases	%
Rigidity of abdominal muscles in right lower abdomen	24	66.6
Tenderness on pressure of right lower abdomen	36	100
Rebounding pain in right lower abdomen	36	100

5. CONDITION OF ACUTE APPENDICITIS CASES AFTER TREATMENT (Only those with complete record included)

Duration	Disappearance of abdominal pain	Normal blood picture	Normal temp.
<24 hours	9	7	12
<2 days	6	4	2
<3 days	5	4	3
<4 days	2	2	2
5-7 days	5	1	–
8 days	1	–	–

6. DURATION OF HOSPITALISATION IN ACUTE APPENDICITIS CASES

Hospital-days	*No. of cases*		
Emergency cases not hospitalised	3		
2 days	4 ⎫		
3 days	3 ⎬ 41.7%		
4 days	6 ⎭		
5 days	8	⎫	
6 days	5	⎬ 78.7%	
8 days	1	⎭	
11 days	1		
12 days	1		
13 days	1		
22 days	1		
	36		

Conclusion: Good results obtained in all the cases. No untoward complications were observed.

C

L. J. Milman, E. D. Tikochinskaia and N. P. Bobrova (Acupuncture Laboratory of the Bechterev Psycho-neurological Institute and the Polyclinic No. 5 in Leningrad)* treated thirty-five cases of physical sexual malfunction, which had proved resistant to ordinary treatment. Twenty-six of these were cured or improved. Of these twenty-six, twenty-four came for a re-check one-and-a-half years later; and of these twenty-four, twenty-one had remained cured or improved.

D

Professor U. G. Vogralik (Gorki Medical Institute) states the following statistics:†

* Russian Acupuncture Conference, Gorki, June 1960.
† Russian Acupuncture Conference, Gorki, 1959.

Disease	No. of Patients	Greatly improved or completely cured	Improved	No change	Treatment continues
Peptic ulceration	48	37	3	2	6
Spastic colitis	5	2	1	1	1
Bronchial asthma	54	3	31	14	6
Thyrotoxicosis (mild & severe)	12	3	6	1	2
Cardiac neurosis	16	0	5	8	3
Angina pectoris	18	7	7	4	—
Angina pectoris (sclerotic)	24	5	11	8	—
Rheumatic coronaritis	2	1	0	1	—
Erythraemia	23	6	11	4	2
Trigeminal neuralgia	13	4	4	1	4
Glaucoma	35	20	4	3	5
	250	88	83	47	

E.

At one time, when I practised acupuncture in hospital, we analysed and published the following results:*

The statistics given on p. 116 refer to 40 consecutive patients seen at the Ear, Nose and Throat Department during the course of a four-year trial period. In each case the main symptom was headache. We chose headache, as this symptom, with some exceptions, is difficult to cure by Western medical methods, while a reasonably permanent cure or considerable alleviation can be achieved by acupuncture in about 80 per cent of the patients treated.

Patients were referred to the Department by their general practitioners or from other departments of the Hospital. They were first seen by one of us (A.H.), and a thorough ENT investigation was made: this included almost invariably

* Felix Mann and Anthony Halfhide, *Medical World,* April 1963.

an X-ray examination of the sinuses. Where the headache was found to be due to ENT disease, such as sinusitis, and amenable to orthodox ENT methods, patients were treated by A.H. without using acupuncture. Such cases are not included in the figures. Other cases excluded were those in which the headache was of minor importance and cases of chronic suppurative otitis media, cranial tumour and so on.

All the patients had been treated for headache without much success by at least two doctors—their GP and a member of the ENT Department. Many of them had been to one or to several other departments of the Hospital as well. Only those cases were treated by acupuncture (by F.M.) in which orthodox medicine had failed or achieved only a slight improvement.

We have not tried to classify the headaches into various types, as the usual definitions are too arbitrary and do not fit in with what we consider to be the important symptoms. Some doctors might have classified about half the patients as having migraine, other doctors, tension headaches, others neuralgia. Two of the headaches were specific—trigeminal neuralgia and supraorbital neuralgia.

The results, as recorded in the table, were as follows: 3 patients (7½ per cent) showed no improvement or aggravation; 5 (12½ per cent) showed moderate improvement; and 32 (80 per cent) were cured or showed considerable improvement. We have adopted this classification as many of the patients have had headache for a large part of their lives and the cause usually goes back several years further. Those very severe cases—those patients who before treatment had spoken of suicide, had stopped work, or were living in a semiconscious state under constant analgesia usually still have an occasional mild headache, and so could be described perhaps as 70 to 99 per cent cured. A few with moderately severe headache still have a very occasional mild one—much as a patient cured of pleurisy may have an occasional pleuritic pain in cold or damp weather.

Some patients, particularly those with severe symptoms of long duration, will probably have a mild recurrence of their

ANALYSIS OF CASES TREATED BY ACUPUNCTURE FOR VARIOUS TYPES OF HEADACHE
AND OTHER SYMPTOMS OR DISEASES

| | | Various types of headache | | | Other symptoms or diseases in the same patient | | | |
Patient	Sex	Duration of headache (years)	Number of treatments	Results	Symptom or Disease	Duration (years)	Number of treatments	Result
J.D.	F	1	1	++	Vertigo	$1\frac{4}{12}$	1	+
M.E.	F	7	1	++				
N.G.	M	5	2	++				
M.H.	M	10	12	+	Asthma	14	15	+
R.L.	M	15	7	++	Lumbago	?	?	++
D.L.	F	2	14	++	Billiousness	2	14	++
L.O	F	2	6	++	Heartburn	2	6	++
B.P.	F	$1\frac{1}{2}$	5	++	Tinnitus	$\frac{8}{52}$	3	++
M.Q.	F	$\frac{1}{2}$	2	++	Asthenia	2	9	++
H.S.	M	8	4	++				
E.S.	F	8	4	++				
E.T.	F	20	8	++	Allergic rhinitis	20	8	+
P.T.	M	4	9	−				
H.T.*	F	3	1					
A.W.	F	20	4	++	Anosmia	2	4	+
H.N.	M	1	14+	+	General debility	1	14+	+
J.T.	M	10	7	++	Allergic rhinitis	10	7	+
D.H.	M	20	4	++	Biliousness	?	7	++
D.B.	M	2	10	++	Asthenia	?	10	+

Patient	Sex				Diagnosis			
P.C.*	M	1	1	++				
R.D.	M	15	3	++				
M.G.	F	1	8	++				
F.E.	M	10	8	++	Hypochondria			
G.C.	F	?1	12	++	This was a case of tri-germinal neuralgia			
A.H.	F	9/12	3	++	This was a case of supraorbital neuralgia			
G.H.	F	6	3	++	Hysterical aphonia	30	6	++
R.H.	F	3	6	++	Allergic rhinitis	3	15	+
M.K.	F	3	15	+	Asthenia			
T.L.	M	9/12	4	++				
K.M.	M	5	2	++				
J.M.	M	4	4	+	Allergic rhinitis	?	4	+
A.N.	F	12	8	++	Biliousness	12	8	++
E.S.	F	3	7	–				
M.S.	F	20	12	++	Allergic rhinitis	20	12	+
A.W.	F	5	3	++	Biliousness	5	3	++
L.P.	F	5	2	–				
E.A.	M	17	6	++	Biliousness	?	5	++
C.L.	F	8	9	++	Anosmia	?	8	++
D.M.	F	1	4	++	Very sleepy	1	4	++
A.M.	M	15	17	+				
V.H.	F	5	11	++				
R.W.	M	10	8	++				

++ cured or considerable improvement
+ moderate improvement
– no improvement or aggravation
* did not continue treatment

headaches after several months or several years of freedom. These can usually be cured in one to three treatments. In the most difficult case there may be several recurrences, each being milder and separated by a longer interval until, in the end, the condition is completely cured, or at least nearly so.

In certain patients with headache due to diseases which cannot be cured by either Western medicine or acupuncture (there are none in this statistical series), it is sometimes possible to alleviate the headache. As the basic condition cannot be cured, constant 'pep up' treatments will be required *ad infinitum*—helpful perhaps but unsatisfactory.

As can be seen from the table, many of the patients had other symptoms or diseases, which were treated at the same time as the headache. (Only the main additional symptom is noted in the statistics.) Mostly the treatment of the other symptoms took the same number of treatments as the headache—thus patient L.O. (7th down) needed a total of 6 treatments to cure both the headache and the heartburn. Sometimes the other symptoms took longer or shorter to cure or alleviate than the headache. Where there was little difference in the number of treatments required to treat both symptoms, the greater number of treatments has been put down under both headings. Where there is a question mark the relevant fact had not been noted in the case history.

XII

THE SCIENTIFIC PROOF

The 'proof' of how medicine worked was explained in medieval Europe by God, the devil and the four humours; in China by Yin, Yang and the five elements. Today the scientific laboratory is the yardstick.

The mechanism of acupuncture is elusive. Nevertheless, I have developed the following theory which I think will soon be generally recognised as the scientific basis of acupuncture—albeit with modifications and considerable clarification in detail.

If a patient has a pain in the head or neck, it may under certain circumstances be alleviated in one second, by putting an acupuncture needle into the correct acupuncture point in the foot. This speed of conduction, from one end of the body to the other, is only possible in the nervous system. It would take about half a minute for the blood to flow such a distance, and the lymphatic circulation is even slower.

Acupuncture is based on the fact that stimulating the skin has an effect on the internal organs and other parts of the body. This nerve reflex may be demonstrated experimentally:

If the skin on the back of rabbits or rats at the level of the lower ribs is stimulated, the circulation of blood in the duodenum is altered.

Likewise in man, if the skin of the upper abdomen is pinched during an operation, the calibre of the blood vessels of the ascending large intestine is altered.

Again, in patients with angina pectoris or in those who have a heart attack, if the trigger areas on the front of the chest are stimulated, prolonged or even complete relief of symptoms arises.

In the above experiments with rats and rabbits, some were done with intact animals using a general anaesthetic, whilst others were performed with the spinal cord transected in the lower neck. In both groups of animals the result of the experiments was the same, showing that the brain and the nerve centres immediately below the brain, are not required in this type of nerve reflex, which is used in acupuncture.

Similar experiments have been made in fish and eels. In an eel which has had its brain destroyed, stimulation of a small area of the skin, causes a constriction of the blood vessels in the subjacent part of the intestine. This is followed by a contraction and later peristaltic movement of the intestine.

If a different part of the skin of the eel was stimulated, the same happened, again in the subjacent part of the intestine. The nearer the head end of the eel the skin was stimulated, the nearer the upper end of the intestine did the changes take place. Likewise in the cod, where stimulation near the fins (equivalent to our arms) caused alterations in the stomach—at the top end of the intestinal tract—whilst stimulation of the tail caused changes at the lower end of the intestine.

This experiment with eel and cod explains the position of certain acupuncture points in man: stimulation of acupuncture points on the chest affect the lungs and heart, stimulation of points on the upper abdomen influences the upper abdominal organs, whilst needling acupuncture points on the lower abdomen affects the bladder and rectum. There is a fine correlation between the organs of the chest and abdomen with the stimulation of the chest, abdomen or back at the correct level.

In another experiment two groups of eel were taken: in one the entire spinal cord was destroyed, whilst in the other it was left intact. When the skin of both groups was stimulated it was found that the blood vessels* of the

* In this and several other experiments, alterations in the flow of blood after stimulating a nerve (i.e. acupuncture) are mentioned. This is only because alterations in the flow of blood are easy to observe in experiments. Many other functions, less easy to observe, but nevertheless there, also alter after acupuncture.

intestine in the former group were constricted whilst in the latter they were dilated. This shows that the spinal cord is necessary in the eel for dilation of blood vessels, whilst the constriction of the blood vessels is mediated by the sympathetic system of nerves.

All the above experiments refer to the type of acupuncture point that has an effect in the same region of the body. If the skin between the shoulder blades is stimulated it has an effect on the lungs and the heart, if the skin over the lower abdomen is stimulated it has an effect on the bladder and lower part of the large intestine. There are though many acupuncture points which are far away from the organ with which they are linked i.e. putting a needle in the foot for a headache. This may be explained by the nervous pathways connecting one end of the body with the other:

One researcher poured boiling water over the hind legs of two unconscious dogs. In one dog the spinal cord had been divided at the level of the bladder, whilst in the other it was intact. In the former dog there was an increased flow of blood in the bladder area, whilst in the other the increased flow also took place in the chest and upper abdomen, thus showing that the spinal cord is needed to transmit the impulse from the leg to the chest.

A similar distant effect is observed in a cat whose mid-brain is divided. If the left ear is pricked then the right hind leg is bent; or if the left hind leg is pricked then the right fore leg is bent. This 'long' reflex takes place within the spinal cord and does not require the sympathetic system.

These experiments may be read in greater detail in my more technical book, Textbook of Acupuncture.

XIII

STRONG REACTORS

Patients Who Respond Well to Acupuncture
Patients Who May Respond Adversely to Normal Doses
of Drugs

There are some patients who respond to acupuncture like magic: an illness which they have had for weeks, months or years may be alleviated or cured within seconds or minutes. Unfortunately this does not happen every day. These magical results occur in perhaps 5 per cent of the population, I call these people Hyper-strong Reactors. Nevertheless, there are many patients who respond very well to acupuncture: I call them Strong Reactors.

Case History. A patient had just been discharged from hospital where she had suffered from meningism (not meningitis) with a temperature of 40°C. When I saw her she felt absolutely awful: she had some difficulty standing, was dizzy, had a continuous headache, disliked the light, had a poor memory and could not think properly. The problem was that on the next day she had to sit her entrance examination for Oxford University, in classics, a difficult subject. I needled four places very gently. She immediately felt some improvement, rested for a couple of hours and then went home. Her mother could not believe her eyes: her daughter came prancing in, saying, 'I feel like a tiger'. She was as if reborn, and passed her university exams.

Response of Strong Reactors to Acupuncture

1. Strong Reactors usually respond immediately and dramatically to acupuncture. Sometimes the response is such that the patients themselves cannot believe it. When I ask how they feel after the treatment there is a long pause–they do not know what to say, for they cannot take in the fact that their symptoms

have gone. They ask me if I am a hypnotist, if I have injected some drug with the acupuncture needle, or how many minutes it will last. This immediate response is not auto-suggestion for, although the patients hoped to get better (most patients visit doctors in that hope!), they thought the response would be slow, for that is what they are used to from orthodox medicine. Quite a number of patients do not really expect any improvement at all, having come to acupuncture as a one-off gamble, after 'real' medicine has failed.

Occasionally a Strong Reactor will only respond hours, days or a week after treatment. The response, however, is greater or very much greater than either patient or doctor expected.

2.(a) Strong Reactors require few needles. Nowadays I frequently needle only one place. They also require a smaller number of treatments.

(b) The needling should be gentle. This means the doctor should use a thin needle, with a smoothly polished surface and a thin, well tapered point. Often the needling is only intracutaneous or subcutaneous and not deeper into the muscles or periosteum. Hence the patient feels very little pain.

(c) The needle or needles should only be left in place for a few seconds before being removed. Most acupuncturists leave the needles sticking in their patients for, say, a quarter of an hour. I never leave the needles in, whether the patient is a Strong Reactor or a Normal Reactor.

It is thus apparent that Strong Reactors receive the dosage of acupuncture that one would otherwise give to a baby. Yet this baby dose has an even greater effect than a normal dose will have in a Normal Reactor.

3. Normal Reactors feel the pin prick of acupuncture locally, perhaps spreading out an inch or two around the needle. Occasionally there may be the radiation of a mild pain or other sensation for a distance of, say, four inches along the limb or part of the body stimulated.

The Strong Reactor, on the other hand, will often have radiation travelling one or two feet, or even from one end of the body to the other. This radiation may sometimes be a mild, but not unpleasant, pain that travels slowly taking, say, three seconds or longer to traverse the length of a limb. More often it is not a pain but a feeling of warmth, or like somebody blowing gently on the skin. Very often it is indescribable, patients just saying it feels like 'something'.

4. Sometimes a Strong Reactor will have a feeling of warmth at the opposite end of the body to the needle prick, particularly in the neck and shoulders, or in the diseased part of the body.

5. The patients may feel slightly relaxed or extremely relaxed. Sometimes they sit still, thinking and doing nothing: day-dreaming in a very pleasant way. Their arm or leg or whole body may feel heavy.

6. Some fall asleep for five minutes, an hour or—more rarely—four hours. When they become drowsy and then sleepy, it is always described as a pleasant sleepiness, not the unpleasant sleepiness of utter exhaustion.

7. A few become euphoric. They feel like a million dollars. They go home, spring clean their house, answer all the unanswered letters, mow the lawn, etc.

Sometimes patients may have a mixture of paragraph 5, 6 and 7: they are relaxed, sleepy and euphoric, all at the same time.

Some suddenly cry for no reason.

Some laugh non-stop.

Case History. A doctor who frequently had migraine came to one of the courses I hold for doctors who wish to learn acupuncture. During the course I needled her very gently. Within a minute or two she started laughing. She continued giggling and spluttering for the next hour until the course finished for the day. She relaxed and dozed here for two hours longer and then caught a taxi home, accompanied by a friend who thought someone should look after her. During the ride she started laughing again: the taxi driver thought she was mad or drunk. At home she laughed for a few hours more until it stopped. The laughter is completely uncontrollable, the patient cannot stop it however embarrassed by it he or she feels. This doctor was cured of her migraine for a whole year, until she needed a second treatment. She is obviously not just a Strong Reactor but a Hyper-strong Reactor.

Some patients may alternate between laughing and crying for a while.

Some patients who have taken drugs, such as marihuana, say that the relaxation, sleepiness or euphoria of acupuncture is similar. They do not, however, become addicted to acupuncture.

Rarely, patients may see colours which are brighter, hear sounds which are clearer and more beautiful, and when they observe nature it acquires a new significance and deeper meaning.

Over-treatment of Strong Reactors

It is extremely important to recognise whether a patient is a Strong Reactor for, if they are given a normal dose of acupuncture, it will be of no benefit.

1. If a Strong Reactor is *moderately* over-treated, he will have a reaction. This is usually a temporary worsening of his present symptoms. If he has migraine, he may have a migraine the same evening as the treatment or the next morning. The migraine may be of normal severity or even worse.

As written previously, a patient may feel relaxed and sleepy after acupuncture. If this lasts for a whole week, the patient has been over-treated.

After the reaction has worn off, which might take a day or a week, the improvement of the patient follows. This improvement is normally as great and long lasting as if the patient had been treated more gently and there had been no reaction. In that sense the reaction has been only an unpleasant but temporary experience, for the end result is the same.

I have the impression from a few patients that occasionally the benefit, after even a mild reaction, is not quite as great as if there had been none. In a few other patients the full benefit of the treatment does not seem to occur unless they have had a reaction.

Occasionally the reaction may not be a temporary worsening of the patient's symptoms, but rather a general feeling of being unwell or a temporary reawakening of symptoms of a different illness a patient had suffered from weeks, months, or years previously.

On other occasions a patient who is moderately over-treated just notices nothing: they do not have a reaction, but neither does their condition improve.

2. If a Strong Reactor is *very much* over-treated, the patient will probably have a reaction, as described in the previous section. After the reaction has worn off, the patient's health just slips back to the state in which it was before acupuncture treatment began; i.e. there is not the delayed improvement one has after moderate over-treatment.

It should be stressed that the reaction is only temporary. One does not have the permanent adverse reaction which on very rare occasions is possible with drugs.

Case History. An organist had suffered from migraine for most of her life. I recognised her to be a Strong Reactor and hence treated her as strongly as I would a five-year-old child. A few hours later she had a severe migraine which lasted several days–longer than usual.

The moment she told me this at the next treatment, I realised I had treated her too strongly and hence treated her on this occasion as a two-year-old child. She telephoned a week later to cancel her next appointment, as again she had been worse straight after the second treatment and she said she could not face it happening again. I begged her to try once more, and, as she knew another patient I had helped, she came.

At the third treatment I treated her as if she were a baby aged six months. From then onwards she improved to such an extent that it transformed her life, enabled her to go away on holiday, etc.

It is thus apparent that one has to recognise not only who is a Strong Reactor, but also to what degree, which is extraordinarily difficult. I will attempt to describe how in the next section.

Normal Reactors can also have a reaction to acupuncture, but it is rare, for in any event, they need a much larger dose.

Some acupuncturists habitually treat all or most of their patients more strongly than I do. They transfix their patients with long, thick, unpolished needles which they twist around till the patient is in pain. Others put an electric current of various intensities through the acupuncture needles for, say, half an hour. To my way of thinking these people are treating their patients incorrectly. They tell me, however, that they get their patients better. Acupuncture is full of contradictions, something one learns to live with.

How to Recognise a Strong Reactor

There is no way one can be 100 per cent sure who is and who is not a Strong Reactor. There is no laboratory test for it. As in many other things in medicine, or life in general, one has to rely on one's judgement.

In reality there is no hard and fast distinction between the two. There is a gradual transition from the Hyper-strong Reactor to the least responsive Normal Reactor. I believe there is no particular concentration of individuals anywhere between the two extremes. There are various methods of distinguishing. The most reliable, yet the most difficult, is the first:

1. If one looks at a Strong Reactor one has the impression they are flexible, somehow not fixed. If a human being were to consist of a hundred pieces of wood, then in the Strong Reactor these hundred pieces would all be interchangeable and variously interlocking. In a Normal Reactor it would be more as if glue had been poured over the hundred pieces of wood, which could no longer be moved about.

One can sometimes tell who is a Strong Reactor on the telephone or from a letter. It is not what is said or written, but rather the tone of voice or how something is described.

2. Strong Reactors may be more sensitive to stimuli than other people. They may look at a cloud and be in absolute raptures about its beauty, whereas the Normal Reactor will merely say it reduces visibility when driving. Strong Reactors may be more intuitive, arriving at conclusions not supported by facts, and yet being often right. A Strong Reactor may sense someone looking at him or her from behind.

Some believe that Strong Reactors are more likely to be volatile or quick thinking. Just as many, however, are phlegmatic, down to earth, slow thinkers.

Being a Strong Reactor has nothing to do with being fat or thin, tall or short, having fine or coarse features, being clever or stupid, having a good or poor education, belonging to a particular race, being rich or poor, being a woman or a man, or being a country or a town dweller. Being a Strong Reactor is not a mental or physical characteristic, rather it is a physiological type, an expression of how someone's physiology ticks and it is this, in turn, which affects the body and the mind, rather than the other way around.

3. Perhaps a third of Strong Reactors respond in a different way to normal doses of drugs (see the next section).

4. Strong Reactors require smaller doses of acupuncture, and when they are needled are more likely to have radiation or other distant effects. They are more likely after treatment to feel relaxed, fall asleep, become euphoric, laugh or cry, as mentioned earlier in this chapter.

5. I have occasionally noticed with a Hyper-strong Reactor that something like 'electricity' passes between the patient and myself.

6. My wife, who is also my secretary, being a Strong Reactor herself, finds it relatively easy to detect other people who are Strong Reactors, on the principle of 'set a thief to catch a thief'. She uses two main methods:

(a) Being a Strong Reactor herself she feels a certain empathy with other Strong Reactors. It is hard to explain, but she feels it.

(b) When she sees a patient she tries to think of another patient who is similar, who somehow reminds her of this patient. It is a little like looking for a very faint family resemblance. Sometimes the patients look physically similar, sometimes not.

As we know how the previous patient responded to acupuncture, we can then deduce how the present patient will probably react.

My wife sees most of the patients who come to our practice when they arrive, or she may have spoken to them on the telephone. We then usually discuss each patient briefly to assess whether and to what degree the patient is a Strong Reactor.

Usually she and I agree, but sometimes not. I have found out that when we disagree she is more often right than I am, and hence now, like all dutiful husbands, I usually do what she says. My wife, however, does not treat the patients as she is not a doctor.

Although we are, of course, not always right, having two people to assess the Strong Reactor or Normal Reactor status of patients is, I think, invaluable. I always tell the doctors who come to the courses I give in acupuncture that they should work with a person who is a Strong Reactor, to see the patients as they come in. Some doctors spend, say, £50000 on x-ray apparatus: in an acupuncture practice a Strong Reactor is worth more.

Sometimes I see a patient who has had acupuncture elsewhere without success. The patient may have heard that I practise acupuncture full time, which very few doctors do in the Western world. Sometimes I can help or cure the patient and sometimes I cannot. If I can, by far the commonest reason is that I have recognised the patient as a Strong Reactor, and have therefore treated him suitably gently.

Within a few weeks of having started my acupuncture practice in 1959, I noticed there were these two types of patient and have developed my acupuncture practice along these lines ever since. I am not aware of this distinction being made by anyone else prior to this anywhere in the world literature on acupuncture.

Subsequently I discovered that the Chinese made a few references to something similar in their very early literature. They distinguish the Fat Type, who should be needled strongly, who is a strong young man who moves slowly, has a big body, wide shoulders, a thick lower lip, dark skin and is a peasant. There is also the Lean Type, who should be needled gently, who is weak, lean, has thin skin, thin lips, white colour, a poor complexion and who belongs to the nobility or scholarly class. It is apparent that this Chinese description is completely different from my own. The Chinese division into Fat and Lean Types could be seen as having a theoretical plausibility but does not, in fact and in my experience, reflect the actual distinction between the different types of reactor.

Patients who may Respond Adversely to Normal Doses of Drugs

Some patients who are Strong Reactors may respond in an unusual manner to drugs. This occurs more amongst the Hyper-strong Reactors than amongst the more usual Strong Reactors. The proportion who react in this way is hard to determine, perhaps, but though I am far from sure, I believe it is about a third of the Hyper-strong and Strong Reactor population.

These patients may feel ill, have side-effects or unusual effects if they take the normal, standard dose of a drug. If these patients take a reduced dose of the same drug they will have the beneficial effect of the drug without the side-effects or the unusual effects.

The issue is complicated as a certain patient may have a different sensitivity to different drugs. For example, a specific individual may require:

1. $\frac{3}{4}$ of the normal dose of drug A.
2. $\frac{1}{2}$ the normal dose of drug B.
3. $\frac{1}{4}$ of the normal dose of drug C.
4. $\frac{1}{10}$ of the normal dose of drug D.
5. The normal dose of drug E.
6. Very rarely–double the normal dose of drug F.

The above is the usual pattern for such patients. There are, however, a few who need half or three-quarters of the dose of nearly all drugs they take–a much simpler state of affairs.

In a chronic disease it is possible to start with a low dose of a drug and then increase the dose gradually until the therapeutic effect is apparent, which is normally at a lower dosage level than the level which may produce side-effects. The whole procedure, however, takes much more time, effort and understanding than merely the prescription of a normal dose.

In acute diseases, where the therapeutic effect is required at once, the past response of the patient can be used as a guide.

All patients have adverse reactions to normal doses of drugs on rare occasions. If this happens frequently, the doctor should always consider carefully if perhaps he is dealing with a Strong Reactor.

There are some patients who have never taken a drug in their whole life and hence it is difficult to assess in this way whether or not they are Strong Reactors. Sometimes these patients have a subconscious fear of or aversion to drugs: they are not really anti-drugs in any conscious way, they just have this feeling. These patients are usually Strong Reactors, whose instinct is right.

I am sure that many of the adverse reactions patients have to drugs occur because most doctors do not distinguish between Strong Reactors and Normal Reactors. If the medical profession and the pharmaceutical industry could solve this problem some ill health would automatically disappear. Doctors would have to learn how to make the extraordinarily difficult diagnosis of a Strong Reactor.

It is even quite possible that some of the drugs which have been withdrawn from use and whose manufacture has been curtailed or stopped would still be in use if the Strong Reactor factor had been taken into account.

XIV

THE LIVER or UPPER DIGESTIVE DYSFUNCTION

I treat the 'liver' virtually every day of my professional life without the patient, even if the patient is a fellow doctor, having realized in the first place that he is suffering from a dysfunction of the 'liver'. Let me explain.

As a young doctor I worked for a while in France where this concept of being livery is part of generally accepted knowledge, known to the whole population and to doctors who practise unorthodox medicine, though to a lesser extent in academic medicine. It is a concept which pervades Southern and Eastern Europe and, I think, North Africa, to a greater or lesser degree, but is little known in Northern Europe or the Anglo-Saxon world. It is as impossible to speak to the French for any length of time without hearing about a *crise de foie* as it is to speak to the English without hearing about the weather.

The ancient Chinese also have a concept of the liver which is largely different from that of both the Anglo-Saxon doctors and the French general population (see my Textbook of Acupuncture, pages 395-403, for a detailed description).

I have taken the French and Chinese ideas and added my own. This chapter is largely based on what patients, who in my practice are not hurried, have told me, added to my observation of what happens after treatment. Simple observation of the patient is not practised often in modern medicine, which feels uncomfortable without laboratory tests, x-rays and biopsies. Modern Western medical books have been of little assistance, as it is a subject which is hardly described, for the simple reason that many doctors do not think the problem even exists!

An analysis of the symptoms associated with the liver will reveal that more than just the liver is involved. The concept actually encompasses all of the upper abdominal organs: liver, gall bladder, the digestive function of the pancreas, stomach, duodenum and possibly jejunum. The syndrome should therefore really be called *upper digestive dysfunction* but as *liver* is the commonly used word, I also use it.

In orthodox medicine the word liver refers to the anatomical liver, which may be affected by diseases such as cirrhosis, cancer or jaundice. This is a completely different concept to the one I am using in this chapter. I think it will be obvious from the context which 'liver' I am referring to.

It is interesting to note that both the sympathetic and parasympathetic nerve supply of all the above-mentioned upper abdominal organs is virtually the same, and also that embryologically they all originate very close to one another.

LIVER SYMPTOMS

There is a huge range of symptoms which may be associated with upper digestive dysfunction, of which the commonest are listed below. It is rare to have all the symptoms mentioned: most people have just one or two. An individual patient may have symptoms in only one group, e.g. a headache; or may have them in two or more groups, e.g. headache and painful periods.

The Feeling of a Mild Hangover

The most typical of all liver symptoms is to wake up in the morning feeling as if one has a very mild hangover. I should think a quarter of the population wakes up a little sleepy and with a slightly thick head. They like to go down to breakfast quietly, read the paper and not talk to anyone. Everything is done in a routine, automated way or, if the breakfast table is differently laid, as at a hotel, the sugar may be thrown away and the wrapping paper put in the coffee cup.

One or two hours later, or possibly only half-way through

the morning, the mist lifts, the mind clarifies, you say good morning with a smile–you are once more a human being.

Headache and Migraine

From my point of view, most patients who have headache or migraine have a dysfunction of the liver. Treating the liver by acupuncture or reducing the intake of rich food or alcohol can alleviate or cure a large number of patients.

Many of these patients may in addition wake up most mornings with a thick head, and have indigestion in the evening after a late and large, rich meal.

A headache or migraine may be precipitated by lack of sleep, too much sleep, worry, anxiety, or a stuffy room. If the liver is treated satisfactorily, these precipitating factors will no longer cause a headache or migraine. If a patient has headache or migraine quite often for no particular reason and, in addition, has them after alcohol or rich food, treatment of the liver by acupuncture will cure the former but only ameliorate the latter.

The Feeling of Having Eaten Twenty Dumplings

It is normal to feel full up and bloated if one has eaten and drunk too much at Christmas Eve and on Christmas Day. If, however, one feels like this after a normal or even a small meal, it is probably due to upper digestive dysfunction. This bloated feeling can extend to the whole body, so that the limbs feel heavy, the mind dull, the abdomen distended with wind. The stools may be slightly soft and sometimes even a little pale.

Peptic Ulcer Type Symptoms

Duodenal ulcers, gastritis, heartburn and related symptoms, may all be part of upper digestive dysfunction.

If these patients eat less rich food, (as described later in this chapter) their symptoms may be reduced or eliminated without any further treatment.

Treatment of the liver by acupuncture may help some of these patients, but not as much as a change of diet. I do not know why acupuncture should be of greater benefit than diet in patients with headache and migraine, whereas in patients with peptic ulcer-type symptoms the diet is of more benefit than acupuncture. It is, however, an observation I have made frequently.

Sometimes these symptoms are precipitated by worry or a shock. I think, though I am not sure, that this does not happen in someone who is not livery and eats the correct diet.

The many drugs which are today available for reducing gastric acidity are very useful. It might be better though if their use were restricted to those few occasions when one cannot avoid a large, rich meal.

The Liver and Mental Symptoms

In orthodox medicine there is a tendency to think that mental diseases have a mental origin, and physical diseases a physical cause.

I think differently: *I think that if there is a disease, or even only a physiological dysfunction of the body, it in turn can cause physical or mental symptoms in variable proportions.*

Pre-menstrual tension has mental symptoms, such as depression or anxiety, and physical symptoms, such as retention of fluid and painful breasts. If the liver is treated by acupuncture, both the physical and mental symptoms of the premenstrual tension are helped, to an equal degree, in quite a high proportion of patients.

I have many patients who have physical as well as mild mental symptoms, both of which, when treated by acupuncture, improve together.

Instead of having a mixture of mental and physical symptoms, some patients have only the extreme of one or the other, which could be expressed as follows:

A physical cause may produce a mental disease
A physical cause may produce a physical disease
A mental cause may produce a mental disease
A mental cause may produce a physical disease

It is because of this interplay between the mind and the body that acupuncture, which is a physical treatment, can help mental conditions. In actual practice, acupuncture only helps the milder mental conditions, the neuroses; the severe mental diseases, the psychoses, are, in my experience, (though some disagree) untreatable.

The type of mental or partially mental symptoms which can be treated via the liver by acupuncture are: pre-menstrual tension, the mental changes some women have with the menopause, and mild depressions. If the depression is so severe that the patient cannot go to work, acupuncture will normally not help.

It is amazing how resistant many in the medical world are to this idea that the mind and body are really one, with one or other side predominating at certain times. I remember many years ago when I was a medical student, being taught that women who had pain at period time were neurotic: when the pill was discovered, which often cures period pain, suddenly women were no longer neurotic! Formerly epileptics were considered mental: when electro-encephalography was discovered and it was shown that epilepsy was a physical disease, these patients were no longer mental!

Case History: For several years a patient had pre-menstrual tension, with mood changes and painful breasts. Life at home and at work was difficult for 10 days each month. Treatment of the liver cured her of both mental and physical symptoms. She needed a 'pep up' treatment once a year for a few years after the initial course of treatments.

Gynaecological Diseases

Many of the milder gynaecological conditions may be helped by acupuncture: painful periods, periods which are too frequent, too infrequent, too heavy or too light. A gynaecologist should first be seen to exclude the possible existence of a more serious condition.

Acupuncture does not help: fibroids, chronic inflammation of the pelvis, vaginal discharge, prolapse of the vagina. Occasionally it may help endometriosis. I do not know if it helps the more recently diagnosed condition of pelvic pain.

Case History: A young lady had painful periods. She did not wish to take the pill as her mother had suffered a thrombosis. She was cured after five treatments, at monthly intervals.

Other Symptoms or Diseases which may be Treated via the Liver

The range of symptoms which may be treated via the liver is vast. In my practice I treat the liver more than anything else; perhaps because I am somewhat livery myself and therefore have a certain empathy with these patients.

Sometimes one can influence the following: lack of energy, acne, mild dizziness, stiff and painful neck, rheumaticky aches and pains, bad taste in the month, occasionally itching skin, and various other 'livery' conditions. A list is given in my Textbook of Acupuncture, pages 395-403.

DIET

Diet can have a major effect on the upper digestive organs, which is what one would expect, as most food is broken down and processed in the upper abdominal organs.

It should be remembered that there is a large variation amongst individuals in dietary matters. There are some who can eat with impunity the forbidden items of a certain diet. There are others who feel ill when eating some of the recommended items.

Some of the symptoms or diseases mentioned in this chapter are best treated by acupuncture, some by diet, but with many a combined approach is better.

Rich Food

Many illnesses and general ill health in Western countries are caused, at least partially, by our Western diet, which is too rich. In poor Third World countries, with their frugal diet, some of the illnesses which we have in the West are a rarity.

Chinese medical books, written 2,000 years ago, give a list of many illnesses which have a greater tendency to occur in wealthy Chinese who eat a rich diet, something a poor peasant could not do. By 'rich' was meant too much fat, oil or sweetness.

The following rich items should be reduced, though not given up completely.

Fats

The fat should be cut off meat and the skin (which is fatty) should be removed from chicken. Meat consumption should be reduced a little, as there is still fat between the meat fibres. Paté and sausages usually contain a high proportion of fat. Game, which runs or flies around in the wild, usually has less fat than farm animals.

Milk contains a lot of fat, as may be seen from looking at a normal bottle of milk. One should, therefore, have skimmed milk, (not semi-skimmed). Also reduce the consumption of butter, cream, cheese, yogurt made from unskimmed milk, etc.

Oils

All vegetable oils should be reduced, particularly olive oil, which is the hardest to digest. Other oils should also be reduced: corn oil, safflower oil, sunflower oil, soya oil, etc. This means a reduction of fried food, mayonnaise, French salad dressing (containing oil), and margarine. Nuts and avocados also contain much oil.

Sugar

Sugar of all types: glucose, dextrose, fructose, sucrose, whether made from cane or beet, white or brown, as well as honey, should be reduced. This means no sugar in tea and coffee; also a reduction in jam, cake, biscuits, ice cream and many soft drinks, squashes and fizzy lemonades. Remember that dried fruit contains more sugar than fresh fruit, which is why it is sweet.

Other items

All forms of alcohol, coffee and chocolate should be reduced drastically. Eggs, smoked salmon and caviar should be eaten only in moderation.

Someone who has eaten too much rich food for many years may no longer notice the effect it has on him, much as an alcoholic may drink several whiskies with little effect whilst a teetotaller may feel the effect of a single whisky. After one has stopped or considerably reduced the consumption of rich food for several months, one may become sensitive to rich food (like a teetotaller to alcohol), so that if one suddenly consumes more than a limited amount, one may feel heavy, over full, slightly headachy, have a thick head, nausea, a dry, bitter or bad taste in the mouth, a feeling like a very mild hangover. The French would call it being 'livery'. It may occur within seconds or twenty-four hours of excessive consumption. This feeling livery is the best guide one can have as to how much rich food one can eat or drink with relative impunity. Some people feel livery with items other than those on this list – these items should be avoided. Others never experience being livery and they cannot use this test.

Gross overeating of any type of food may have the same effect as eating moderately too much rich food.

Some people are hypersensitive to certain foodstuffs, (nothing to do with rich food), chemical additives, etc. This may cause a large variety of illnesses or symptoms, and a cure depends on excluding the offending item or items. This is not the same as the intolerance of rich food mentioned above, though both conditions may co-exist.

TEXTBOOK OF ACUPUNCTURE

Section 1
SCIENTIFIC ASPECTS OF ACUPUNCTURE

Nowadays, the effect acupuncture has on certain diseases can be explained, at least partially, by the spinal and autonomic nerve reflexes between the skin and the viscera - as described in this section. The acupuncture points are reflexly tender areas such as McBurney's point, the meridians are in a few ways related to the dermatomes, whilst the laws of acupuncture can be better explained in terms of ordinary physiology.

This section is almost certainly the first work of a scientific nature to be written on acupuncture.

It shows that the traditional 'acupuncture point' does not exist, that the 'meridians' are imaginary lines, and that the 'laws of acupuncture' are largely mythical. The reader will see that the traditional theoretical foundation of acupuncture is mostly incorrect. Despite this, acupuncture works in a reasonable proportion of patients who have diseases amenable to acupuncture. There are 44 drawings.

Section 2
ACUPUNCTURE: THE ANCIENT CHINESE ART OF HEALING

This book describes the basic principles and laws of acupuncture.

There are chapters on Yin and Yang, the five elements, the details of pulse diagnosis, the laws of acupuncture, Qi — the energy of life, preventive medicine, the cause of disease, the categories of acupuncture points, and statistics. The book is liberally spiced with old Chinese quotations as illustrations of the theory and practice of this 'ancient art'.

It is written as a traditional Chinese book, though in a manner such that the Westerner may understand it. There are 56 drawings and numerous tables.

Section 3
THE MERIDIANS OF ACUPUNCTURE

The course, function and symptomatology of the fifty-nine meridians, which constitute the basis of classical Chinese Acupuncture, are portrayed in detail:

The 12 meridians and their branches

The   8 extra meridians   The 12 divergent meridians
The 12 muscle meridians   The 15 connecting meridians

In addition, the traditional Chinese physiology and pathology of the twelve main groups of internal organs are described. These conceptions have been correlated with the ideas of Western scientific medicine wherever possible. There are 53 full page drawings.

Section 4
THE TREATMENT OF DISEASE BY ACUPUNCTURE

Part I Function of Acupuncture Points
In this part the acupuncture points themselves are taken as the point of departure. Each acupuncture point is listed separately and a full account of the symptoms and diseases that may be influenced by stimulating a specific point is given, following the classical Chinese pattern.

Part II The Treatment of Disease
In this part, by contrast, the departure point is the disease. The majority of diseases amenable to acupuncture are tabulated with the corresponding acupuncture points used for treatment. This part is again divided into two sections: the first is based entirely on Chinese sources, whilst the second describes the experience of the author and other European doctors.

ATLAS OF ACUPUNCTURE

The acupuncture points and meridians are shown in relation
to the bones and skeletal musculature, stressing those anatomical features which are necessary for quick and accurate
anatomical localisation. The format has been designed to
facilitate easy reference in a book of manageable size.

INDEX